THE HASHIMOTO'S
COOKBOOK AND
ACTION PLAN

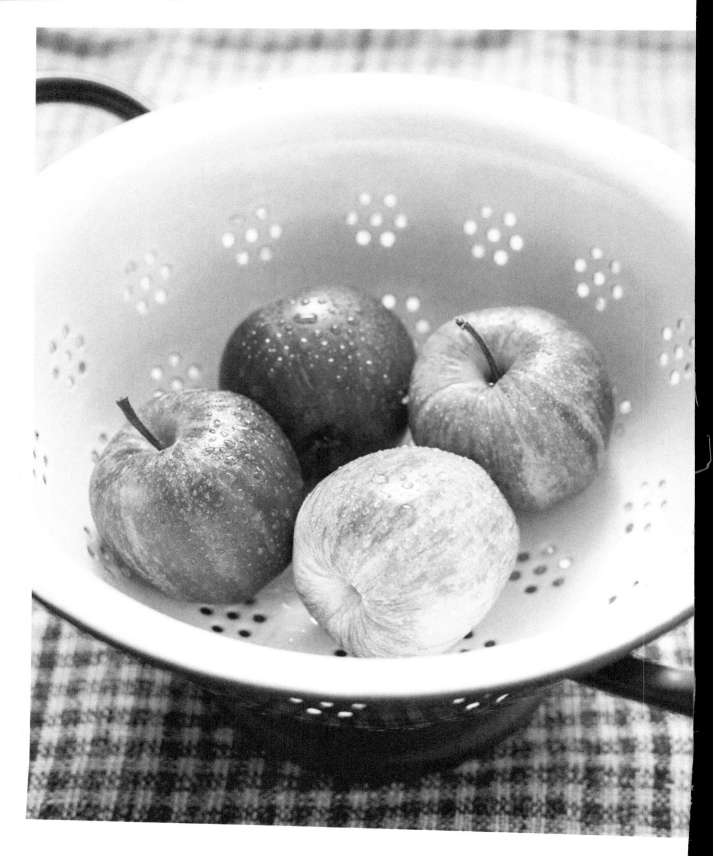

THE HASHIMOTO'S COOKBOOK AND ACTION PLAN

31 DAYS TO ELIMINATE TOXINS AND RESTORE THYROID HEALTH THROUGH DIET

KAREN FRAZIER

in collaboration with

ROCKRIDGE
PRESS

Cover photographs © (front) George Seper/Stockfood; (back, left to right) George Seper/Stockfood; Kristin Duvall/Stocksy; Jacqueline Miller/Stocksy; Andre Baranowski/Stockfood; Rua Castilho/Stockfood.

Interior photographs © Darren Muir/Stocksy, pg. 2; Kristin Duvall/Stocksy, pg. 6; Danil Nevsky/Stocksy, pg. 8; Andre Baranowski/Stockfood, pg. 14; Rua Castilho /Stockfood, pg. 38; Oliver Brachat/Stockfood, pg. 60; Jacqueline Miller/Stocksy, pg. 72; Clinton Hussey/Stockfood, pg. 94; George Seper/Stockfood, pg. 112; Emily Brooke Sandor Photography/Stockfood, pg. 130; Gräfe & Unzer Verlag / Lang, Coco/Stockfood, pg. 142; Gräfe & Unzer Verlag / Grossmann.Schuerle/Stockfood, pg. 166; Sporrer/Skowronek/Stockfood, pg. 184; Lawren Lu/Stocksy, pg. 224. All other photos Shutterstock and iStock.

ISBN: Print 978-1-62315-583-4 | eBook 978-1-62315-584-1

FIVE TIPS
TO TREAT HASHIMOTO'S
THROUGH DIET

1 **Eat real food.** Eating healthy, whole foods without chemicals and artificial ingredients is the first step to healing your body. This includes produce, herbs and spices, animal proteins, and eggs.

2 **Avoid processed foods and sugar.** A good basic rule when shopping for your food is this: Buy ingredients, not products. Processed foods are industrialized products with long lists of ingredients. Instead of foods with long ingredient lists that your ancestors wouldn't recognize, buy and cook with simple ingredients.

3 **Avoid chemicals.** Skip foods that contain additives, preservatives, artificial colors, genetically modified ingredients, and pesticides.

4 **Know your personal triggers.** This plan will help you identify the foods that trigger your Hashimoto's symptoms. Once you have identified your trigger foods, you will need to eliminate them permanently to avoid flare-ups of your symptoms.

5 **Realize this is a lifestyle change and not a temporary diet.** The right mindset is key in helping your Hashimoto's. This is about making changes to your lifestyle so that your body can finally feel better. When you undo those changes, it is very likely your symptoms will return over time. Manage your expectations from the start, and remember that no food item is more important than your health.

CONTENTS

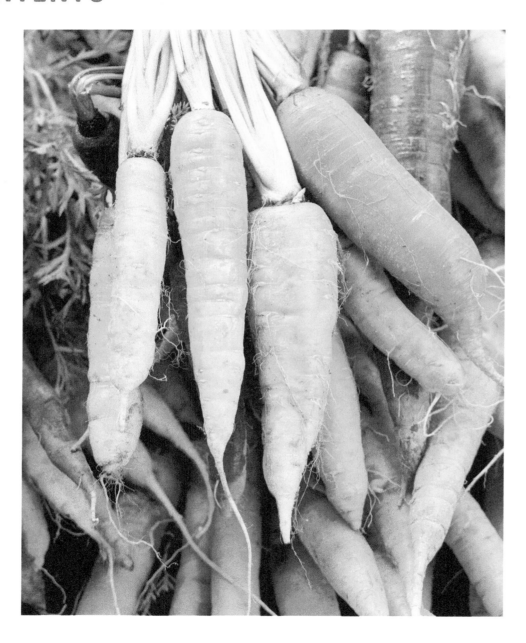

INTRODUCTION

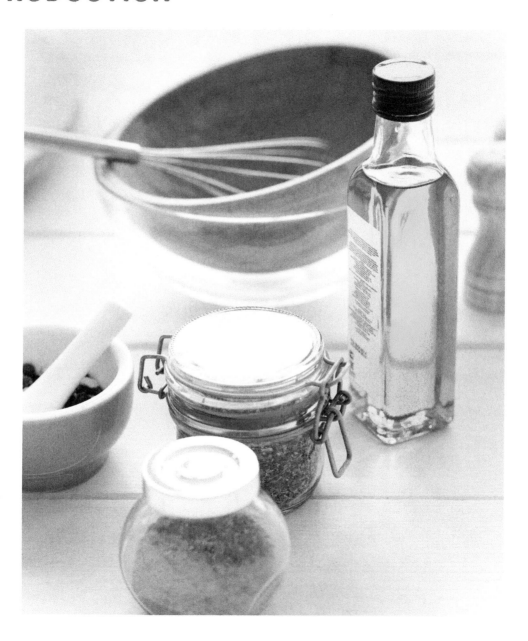

HOW MY DIET HELPED MY HASHIMOTO'S

I can still remember when I first realized something was wrong. I was twenty-three years old and very active. Along with teaching twelve aerobics classes a week, I was also a competitive bodybuilder and a personal trainer. When I wasn't at the gym, I was hiking; jogging; playing tennis, racquetball, and soccer; and bicycling. My whole life was about getting out and moving. I was a bundle of energy.

Then, one morning I woke up and it was like a switch had flipped. All of a sudden I was exhausted. I had no energy. My brain was foggy, my hair was falling out, and I began to struggle with my weight. Within about six months, I went from a lean one hundred twenty-five pounds to over two hundred pounds and climbing. I was cold all the time. My body ached constantly; I felt as if I had been hit by a bus.

I went to see my doctor, who asked me, "Why are you getting so fat?"

When I told him I was eating a low-calorie diet and still exercising as much as I could, he suggested I was delusional or that I was flat-out misrepresenting my activity level and the amount of food I ate. I wasn't.

It took me twenty years to finally get a diagnosis of Hashimoto's thyroiditis—or autoimmune thyroid disease. By that time, my weight had ballooned to over three hundred pounds and I was constantly exhausted. I no longer had the energy to be even slightly active. I was in constant pain, and it took everything I had just to get out of bed every morning, keep the house clean, and do my work. I had migraines about fifteen days out of every month, and my period had become so heavy and painful, I couldn't leave the house when I had it.

When I received my Hashimoto's diagnosis I cried, because I was so relieved that I would finally be able to do something about my health. My doctor prescribed natural desiccated thyroid medication, an extract made from the actual thyroid gland of a pig.

The thyroid medication helped a little, but not nearly as much as I thought it would. I lost a little weight, but my body seemed to still hold on to it. I had a little more energy, but not much. Still, the Hashimoto's diagnosis was a start, and it served as the impetus to discover more about my health. A few years after my diagnosis, following some further medical testing, I discovered I had two more conditions that often go hand in hand with Hashimoto's: celiac disease, which is an autoimmune gluten intolerance, and a casein/dairy allergy. My doctor strongly urged me to cut dairy and gluten out of my life, but I just couldn't imagine my life without bread or cheese. My attempts were half-hearted and short-lived.

Then, at the age of fifty-one, my husband had a mild heart attack. That was a wake-up call for both of us. I delved deep into nutritional research, an interest of mine since the days when I was a personal trainer. Given what I read in medical and nutrition journals, a modified Paleo diet seemed to be the best possible approach to eating. We adopted the Paleo approach to eating from the moment my husband returned home from the hospital, and never turned back.

Within a few weeks, I felt like an entirely different person. My husband and I often joked that I've never been warm a day in my life, and all of a sudden I needed fewer bed covers and fewer sweaters. I was warm! What I thought was irritable bowel syndrome—it involved multiple trips to the bathroom every day—went away completely. My brain fog cleared up. I had so much energy, I almost didn't know what to do with myself. My migraines dissipated. I started having manageable periods. My skin cleared right up. I began losing weight at a really fast clip: about three pounds per week. The chronic, constant pain in my neck, back, and hips became a thing of the past. I was able to get off the medication I'd taken for the past five years for gastroesophageal reflux disease (GERD) without any lingering symptoms. I truly felt—and continue to feel—like a new person.

A change in diet enabled me, at the age of forty-nine, to feel like the young woman I was more than twenty-five years ago, just before the switch flipped and changed everything. It's nice to have her back.

When I was struggling with the symptoms caused by my Hashimoto's, I didn't have a dietary template to follow. This book contains such a plan. For thirty-one days, you will not have to think about what to eat—the meal plans, the shopping lists, and the recipes are all provided. By following the plan, you will give your body a chance to heal. When the month is over, there is guidance for how to reintroduce certain types of foods back into your diet. During this period, which may take several weeks, you can customize the Hashimoto's diet so that it works for your body's own unique needs.

With all my experimentation over the years, one of the things I've come to understand is this: No matter which dietary approach you choose, if the food doesn't taste good, the diet will be difficult to follow. That's why this book is packed with tasty recipes. It allows you to eat foods that are so delicious, you won't even miss the foods you've eliminated. That way, you're giving yourself the best possible chance to heal your body.

Eating this way worked wonders for me, and it is intended to ease some of your Hashimoto's symptoms as well. I hope that within the next thirty-one days, you will discover a new, energetic, and healthy you.

PART

1

HASHIMOTO'S DISEASE AND DIET

CHAPTER ONE

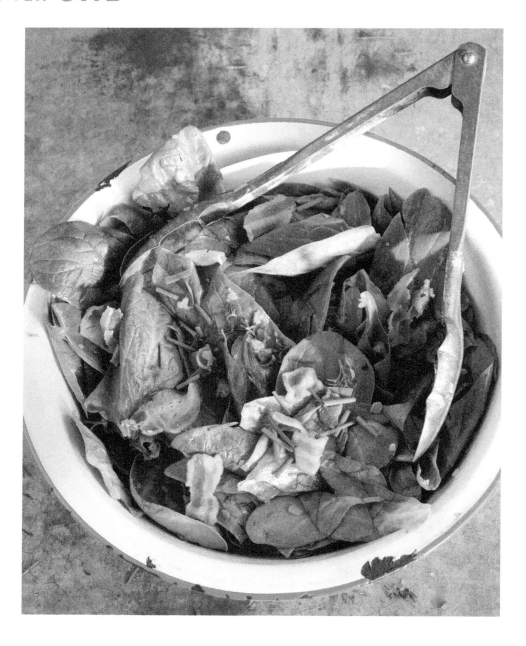

UNDERSTANDING HASHIMOTO'S

Congratulations on taking a big step in managing your Hashimoto's thyroiditis. This book may provide one of the keys to the health reset you need. Whether you've struggled with Hashimoto's for years or have recently received a diagnosis, chances are that if you have Hashimoto's, you've spent some time not feeling very well. I know I did. While the symptoms of this autoimmune disorder vary from person to person, they often diminish quality of life. Making the dietary changes recommended in this book may help control or eliminate some or all of these symptoms.

Your doctor has probably prescribed medication to help control your Hashimoto's, and that is a great first step in managing the condition. He or she may have recommended other lifestyle interventions as well, such as exercise. What many people (including some doctors) may not realize, however, is that changing your diet can play a huge role in controlling your Hashimoto's symptoms.

The information in this cookbook will help you address the dietary component of managing Hashimoto's disease. It is not intended as a substitute for quality medical care. Instead, use it in addition to your health care provider's recommendations.

If you have never attempted dietary change as part of your Hashimoto's self-care plan, or if you've tried to make dietary changes but have found it difficult to do so, this book is for you. It provides meal plans and recipes that remove foods from your diet that may be exacerbating your symptoms, while adding nutritionally dense, delicious foods that support vibrant good health. The recipes are delicious, and the meal plan template is easy to follow. This combination of tasty food and a step-by-step guide to eliminating and reintro-ducing foods provides you with a blueprint for success.

If you've struggled for years with lingering Hashimoto's symptoms despite your medication, or if you are newly diagnosed and seeking to make the best choices to support your journey to health, this book will put you on the right track. With simple concepts and an easy-to-apply plan, *The Hashimoto's Cookbook and Action Plan* will put you on the path to better health.

So You Have Hashimoto's

Hashimoto's disease is also called Hashimoto's thyroiditis, chronic lympho-cytic thyroiditis, autoimmune thyroiditis, and autoimmune thyroid disease. According to the National Endocrine and Metabolic Disease Information Service (NEMDIS), Hashimoto's is the most common cause of hypothyroid-ism in the United States.

Hashimoto's is an autoimmune disease in which the body's immune system attacks the thyroid gland. This leads to chronic inflammation, as well as impaired ability to produce the thyroid hormones necessary for good health. Since the proper balance of thyroid hormones is essential for maintaining a healthy metabolism, the result of improper thyroid hormone function is often a reduction in the body's metabolic rate.

What Causes Hashimoto's?

Autoimmune thyroid disease has a number of possible causes. The US Depart-ment of Health and Human Services (HHS) Office of Women's Health notes that Hashimoto's disease is about seven times more common in women than in men. The most common onset of the disease occurs in middle age.

Hashimoto's disease may occur in clusters along with other autoimmune conditions. A study of more than three thousand people with Hashimoto's disease that appeared in the *American Journal of Medicine* showed that other autoimmune conditions were clustered with Hashimoto's thyroiditis in 14.3 percent of the cases. While the most common disease in the cluster was rheumatoid arthritis, other diseases with statistically significant clus-tering with Hashimoto's included lupus, pernicious anemia, celiac disease, Addison's disease, and vitiligo. In my case, I have the cluster of celiac disease,

Hashimoto's, and a dairy allergy. You may have this cluster, a different cluster, or you may have Hashimoto's alone.

Along with autoimmune clusters, several other characteristics may play a role in Hashimoto's thyroiditis. Potential causes include:

- *Genetics:* The Johns Hopkins Medical Institutions note that the tendency to develop any autoimmune disease is inherited. People who are closely related are more likely to develop the same or related autoimmune diseases.

- *Standard American Diet (SAD):* According to the Arizona Center for Advanced Medicine, SAD has contributed significantly to a rise in autoimmune conditions. Along with being a pro-inflammatory diet, SAD also supports a poor balance of gut bacteria and leads to leaky gut (see the box on page 20), which has been implicated in autoimmune diseases such as Hashimoto's thyroiditis.

- *Pregnancy:* According to NEMDIS, 4 to 10 percent of women experience postpartum hypothyroidism within a year of giving birth. In many cases, this has an autoimmune component. While some women return to normal after a few months, others sustain damage to the thyroid that leads to a lifetime of autoimmune hypothyroidism. In women who've experienced it, postpartum hypothyroidism is likely to recur with every pregnancy.

- *Too much iodine:* The HHS Office of Women's Health suggests that a diet containing too much iodine can trigger Hashimoto's thyroiditis. Since table salt in the United States often contains added iodine and many processed foods contain table salt, consuming too much of these foods may be a trigger for Hashimoto's thyroiditis.

How Hashimoto's Feels

The symptoms of Hashimoto's vary widely depending on the person. While there are some common symptoms, many people with Hashimoto's report an array of strange symptoms that resolve as they regain dietary and medical control of their condition. These symptoms may be mild or severe, and they may change throughout the course of the disease. For many, the symptoms are severe enough to significantly reduce quality of life. While medication may help reduce or eliminate some of these symptoms, many people note that they persist even after they begin taking medication.

Some of the more common symptoms reported include:

- *Cold intolerance:* A sluggish metabolism leads to one of the most commonly reported symptoms associated with hypothyroidism. You may feel chilled all the time, regardless of the ambient temperature of the room.

- *Fatigue:* Many people with Hashimoto's report chronic fatigue. This may range from mild tiredness even after a good night's sleep to constant sheer exhaustion. The fatigue may make it difficult to go about the tasks of daily life. You may feel especially fatigued after exercising or exertion. The Mayo Clinic states that this fatigue arises due to slowed metabolic processes.

- *Cognitive issues:* This is most commonly described as brain fog, and that is exactly how it feels. You feel as if you are trying to think from beneath a dense layer of fog. It occurs because the brain needs thyroid hormones to function. In the absence of sufficient thyroid hormones, thinking becomes more difficult.

- *Menstrual problems:* Because Hashimoto's affects hormone levels throughout the body, many women report having moderate to severe menstrual problems. These often include irregular, extremely heavy, and painful periods.

- *Aches and pains:* According to the Mayo Clinic, people with Hashimoto's thyroiditis report chronic mild, moderate, or severe aches and pains in muscles and joints. Hormonal deficiencies lead to these aches and pains, which may occur throughout the body. Common locations include the hips, shoulders, wrists, and back. For some, the pain is constant. For others, the pain comes and goes, varying in intensity.

- *Bowel problems:* Hypothyroidism slows the movement of the bowel tract, leading to constipation. While the most common bowel problem noted with Hashimoto's is constipation, in some cases, people with Hashimoto's report having alternating bouts of constipation and diarrhea. The latter is more likely to occur when celiac disease or irritable bowel syndrome (IBS) occur in an autoimmune cluster along with Hashimoto's.

- *Weight gain:* A slowed metabolism leads to gaining unexplained weight, which is one of the more emotionally difficult symptoms of Hashimoto's thyroiditis that many people experience. Many gain the weight regardless of diet and exercise habits, which is frustrating and demoralizing.

- *Depression:* Hashimoto's patients also report symptoms of depression and anxiety, such as prolonged feelings of sadness, hopelessness, and anxiety attacks. According to WebMD, these feelings of depression most likely result from the imbalance of hormones brought about by the disease.

TESTS TO REQUEST

If you suspect you have Hashimoto's thyroiditis, you may need to advocate for yourself with your medical doctor. It took me the better part of twenty years of self-advocacy to finally get the tests I needed for my Hashimoto's.

While many doctors will perform a basic blood test for hypothyroidism, they sometimes fail to request a full panel that will give them all the information they need. When talking to your doctor about hypothyroidism, request the following tests.

TSH: This test measures your body's thyroid-stimulating hormone, which your pituitary gland produces. According to MedlinePlus, normal TSH ranges are from .4 to 4.0. High levels may indicate hypothyroidism, while low levels may indicate hyperthyroidism or a pituitary problem.

Free T4: T4 is thyroxine, the main hormone your thyroid produces. The normal range is 4.5 to 11.2. Low levels may indicate hypothyroidism, while high levels may indicate hyperthyroidism.

Free T3: T3 is triiodothyronine, another thyroid hormone. The normal range for T3 is 100 to 200. Low T3 may indicate an underactive thyroid, while high T3 may indicate an overactive thyroid.

Anti-thyroglobulin and anti-thyroid peroxidase antibodies: High levels of these antibodies suggest damage to the thyroid, as you would find in Hashimoto's thyroiditis.

In *The Immune System Recovery Plan*, Susan Blum, MD, notes that if TSH is over 3.0, free T4 is under 1.0, and free T3 is under 2.6, you may have signs of damage from thyroid disease.

GO WITH YOUR GUT

It is difficult to have a discussion about autoimmune disease without talking about leaky gut syndrome. Many practitioners have started to view leaky gut syndrome as a primary culprit in—or at least a contributor to—autoimmune disease. While conventional medicine has resisted the idea of leaky gut syndrome, Dr. Andrew Weil, founder and director of the Arizona Center for Integrative Medicine at the University of Arizona, notes that a growing body of evidence suggests the veracity of this theory.

According to Dr. Weil, SAD causes damage to the intestinal walls, which over time become more permeable. This permeability allows incompletely digested large molecules of food to leak through the walls of the gut into the body and bloodstream. These molecules may contain toxins, undigested proteins, and wastes that are not meant to be in the bloodstream. Since the body does not recognize these particles as beneficial and detects that they may be harmful, it launches an immune system attack on them, leading to inflammation and an autoimmune response. As ongoing exposure occurs, the body begins to attack its own tissue, much as it does in the case of Hashimoto's thyroiditis.

As research continues into leaky gut syndrome, many have recommended healing protocols to help improve intestinal permeability. The SAD fosters the growth of harmful bacteria in the gut, which contributes to its permeability. Incorporating beneficial bacteria in the form of probiotics and fermented foods can help recolonize the gut with beneficial bacteria, which crowd out the harmful bacteria. This, in turn, helps to decrease the permeability of the gut, lessening the autoimmune response and allowing the body to begin to heal.

Another consideration with your gut is bacterial colonization. When you're healing your gut, making sure you colonize it with healthy bacteria can help speed up the process. That's why so many health care providers recommend probiotics for people seeking to heal autoimmune conditions. You can include more probiotics in your diet by eating naturally fermented foods, such as raw sauerkraut (you can find it at the health food store), as well as by taking a quality probiotic supplement.

Hashimoto's FAQ

Should I stop eating table salt?

In the United States, food manufacturers enrich table salt with iodine and call it iodized salt. A little bit of iodine is actually supportive of the thyroid. Too much, however, can do damage. Table salt is also processed and stripped of much of its mineral content. Therefore, if you can afford it, sea salt or Himalayan pink salt, which maintain their mineral content, are best for this diet. If money is an issue, you can also try non-iodized or kosher salt.

Do I have to change the way I eat forever to control my symptoms?

The following chapters will outline a plan that takes you through the next thirty-one days. After that, you will gradually reintroduce foods to see which ones cause your symptoms. You may not need to follow the strictest form of the diet for the rest of your life, but if you would like to see a continued reduction of symptoms, you will very likely need to follow a modified form of it.

How long will it take for me to feel better?

Everyone is different, but some people begin to notice a reduction in symptoms within a few days. Some people may need a few weeks or longer. Following the plan exactly will help you feel better faster. With this plan, having even a taste of something not allowed may be enough to trigger your symptoms.

Will I be able to stop taking my thyroid medication?

This is something you should monitor closely with your endocrinologist. Tell your doctor you are following this plan, and ask him or her to monitor your thyroid hormones. Don't make decisions about your medication without your doctor.

CHAPTER TWO

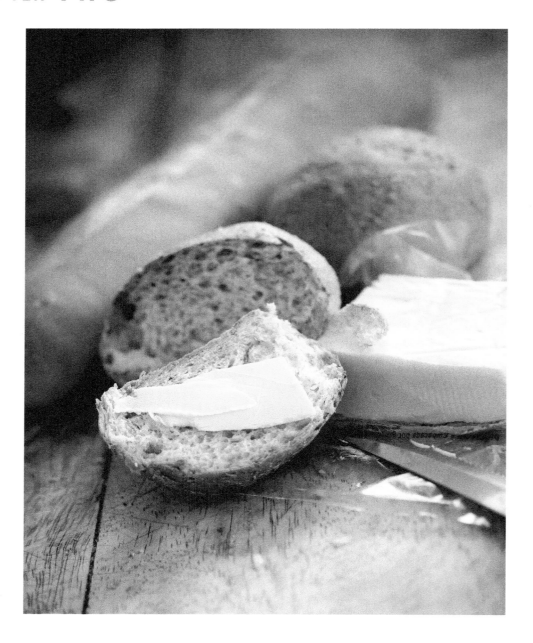

THE DIET CONNECTION

Hippocrates famously said, "Let food be thy medicine and medicine be thy food." He was right. What you eat is tremendously important to your health. If you take a look at the declining health of populations following the Standard American Diet, it becomes immediately obvious that this way of eating does not promote good health.

There is another way, however. Over the past several years, many people have decided to replace the chemicals, sugar, and empty nutrition of highly processed foods with nutrient-dense, wholesome, flavorful foods. Many of these people have found that the symptoms they once experienced, which they believed were just a byproduct of modern life, went away when their diets changed.

This has been especially true for people with autoimmune conditions who began following a diet called the Autoimmune Protocol (AIP), a Paleo-style diet that provides nutritious foods while promoting gut healing and reducing inflammation. The plan and recipes in this book are a modified version of the AIP diet.

The Paleo diet takes a simple approach to food. It is an eating lifestyle based on that of our human ancestors. People on the Paleo diet eat foods that most closely approximate what our ancestors ate: seasonal whole foods that can be hunted or gathered.

Think back to one of your caveman ancestors, Thag. Imagine Thag coming out of his cave to find food. You notice he has a spear in his hands. Thag's wife follows closely with a basket. Neither will head out to the grocery store. Instead, Thag and his wife will hunt for large and small game. They will gather the eggs, fruits, vegetables, herbs, nuts, and seeds that are seasonably available. This is their diet.

Know Your Dietary Triggers

Today's standard diet contains a large number of foods Thag wouldn't have recognized as edible. Unfortunately, many of these modern foods contribute to inflammation and autoimmune responses in your body. Human biology is unique from person to person, however, so everyone is different. The foods that trigger inflammation in one person may be perfectly fine in another. The goal with this diet, then, is to eliminate all possible triggers and then add them back in one at a time to identify the foods that trigger your symptoms. The possible trigger foods are described below.

Gluten

Gluten is a sticky protein found in wheat, rye, triticale, and barley. Many people have difficulty processing gluten, which can lead to a number of uncomfortable symptoms. At the most severe end of the spectrum, gluten-sensitive people have celiac disease, a condition in which consuming gluten causes severe damage to the intestine, making it difficult for them to absorb nutrients from food. At the other end of the spectrum are people with non-celiac gluten intolerance, or gluten sensitivity. These people may experience symptoms from gluten such as inflammation and irritable bowel syndrome.

According to Celiac Central, the online home of the National Foundation for Celiac Awareness, about 1 percent of the population has celiac disease. People with celiac disease cannot eat even a trace of gluten or they will experience intestinal damage. People with non-celiac gluten intolerance may be able to tolerate very small amounts of gluten.

Celiac Central also notes that a large number of people have an innate immune response to gluten. While recent research suggests that some of this may be related to an intolerance to a certain type of carbohydrates called FODMAPs, it is important to note that all gluten grains are actually FODMAPs.

With so many people potentially sensitive to gluten in foods, this diet eliminates them completely. After the thirty-one days, you can add them back in to see if you react to them. Meanwhile, when shopping, read labels carefully. Gluten hides in a number of foods.

Grains

Early humans did not cultivate and eat grains. According to an article in the journal *Nutrients,* consumption of cereal grains can result in chronic inflammation and the development of autoimmune disease in some people. On this protocol, you will avoid grains (many of which also contain gluten) for the first thirty-one days. Then you can introduce one grain at a time over your reintroduction period, to establish which grains cause your unique symptoms.

Avoid all sources of gluten and all grains, including:

Baked goods	Crackers	Pasta
Barley	Croutons	Quinoa
Beer	Farro	Rice
Bread crumbs	Flour	Rye
Buckwheat	Gravy	Soups and stews
Bulgur	Matzo	(unless you know
Cereal	Millet	all the ingredients)
Condiments	Muesli	Soy sauce
(highly processed)	Oats (processed	Spelt
Corn	in a facility that	Wheat
Couscous	contains gluten)	

Dairy Products

Dairy products contain casein, a milk protein that is very similar in structure to gluten. They also contain lactose, a sugar that many people find very difficult to digest. Since dairy is such a common autoimmune trigger, due to both lactose and casein, you will need to eliminate it completely. Then you can try adding it back in during the reintroduction phase of the diet and see how you respond.

You'll notice that margarine is included on this list, even though there are dairy-free margarines. Margarines contain industrial seed oils and hydrogenated fats, as well as other chemicals, so they are not allowed on this diet. Also, many "non-dairy" margarines contain casein.

Avoid all dairy products, including:

Butter	Heavy cream	Rennet
Buttermilk	Ice cream	Sour cream
Casein	Lactose	Whey
Cheese	Margarine	Whipped cream
Cottage cheese	Milk	Yogurt
Custard	Pudding	

Legumes

Starchy legumes, such as kidney beans and lentils, are FODMAPs, and they also contain lectins, which are also found in grains. As noted in the journal *Nutrients*, lectins contribute to inflammation, gut permeability, and auto-immune disease.

Avoid all legumes, including:

Beans	Chickpeas	Peanuts
Cashews	Lentils	Peas

Please note the presence of peanuts and cashews on this list. While many people consider them nuts, peanuts are actually legumes, while cashews are technically seeds (although they can still cause problems). Please note also that green beans are a vegetable and not a legume, so you can eat them on this plan.

Corn

In the documentary *King Corn*, the producers note that nearly every food in the Standard American Diet contains corn. Corn is widely processed into a number of ingredients in processed foods, from cornstarch and cooking oil to high-fructose corn syrup. According to the USDA, more than 80 percent of the corn crops in the United States are genetically modified for herbicide and pes-ticide tolerance. Since genetically modified crops became commonplace only in 1996, the long-term health effects of such modification on the people and animals who eat this corn remain unknown. Additionally, corn is a grain and a FODMAP. Therefore, you need to avoid it while following this plan.

Avoid corn and corn products, including:

Corn bread	Cornstarch	Polenta
Corn cereal	High-fructose corn	Popcorn
Corn chips	syrup	Tortillas and
Corn syrup	Maltodextrin	tortilla chips
	Masa harina	

Soy

The USDA notes that more than 90 percent of the soy crops grown in the United States are genetically modified, and many processed foods contain highly processed forms of this ingredient. Also, soy is a legume and a FODMAP, both of which can be detrimental to people with autoimmune conditions. Of special interest to people with Hashimoto's disease are soy's goitrogenic properties. Goitrogens are substances that inhibit thyroid function.

Avoid all soy and soy products, including:

Anything with ingredients such as soy lecithin or hydrolyzed soy protein	Edamame	Tamari
	Miso	Tempeh
	MSG (monosodium glutamate)	Teriyaki sauce
		Textured vegetable protein (TVP)
Bean curd	Natto	Tofu
Bean sprouts	Soy sauce	
	Soybean oil	

Some Fish

You don't need to avoid fish. In fact, fish can be wonderful because it contains healthy omega-3 fatty acids. However, some fish is quite high in mercury content, and these should be avoided. According to the Natural Resources Defense Council, the fish with the most mercury include:

Ahi tuna	Farmed salmon (wild-caught is okay)	Orange roughy
Albacore tuna		Shark
Bigeye tuna		Swordfish
Bluefish	Grouper	Tilefish
Chilean sea bass	Mackerel	Yellowfin tuna
	Marlin	

Nightshades

Some people have a sensitivity to nightshades, which can cause problems with inflammation, leaky gut, and autoimmune disease. While not all the recipes in this book are nightshade-free, none of the recipes on the thirty-one-day plan contain them. If you notice symptoms during the reintroduction phase after consuming a recipe that contains nightshades, eliminate them completely from your diet. Note that sweet potatoes are not part of the nightshade family, and you can eat them on this diet. Nightshades include:

Cayenne	Paprika	Tobacco
Chile peppers	Potatoes (purple,	Tomatillos
Chili powder	red, white)	Tomatoes
Eggplant	Sweet peppers	

Nuts and Seeds

Because some people with autoimmune disease experience problems with nuts and seeds, they are not included in recipes for the first thirty-one days. Tree nuts are one of the most common allergies people have. If you are allergic to nuts, or if you experience symptoms after eating nuts and seeds, avoid the recipes that contain them. Common nuts and seeds include:

Almonds	Flaxseed	Pumpkin seeds
Brazil nuts	Hazelnuts	Sesame seeds
Chestnuts	Macadamia nuts	Sunflower seeds
Chia seeds	Pecans	Walnuts

Other Dietary Triggers

While the preceding lists cover the main categories, there are some other dietary triggers you'll need to avoid as well.

Sugars

According to Marcelle Pick, a nurse practitioner and founder of Women to Women, a women's health clinic and information source, consuming sugar can increase or ignite the body's inflammatory processes. This diet eliminates all forms of added sugar, including:

Agave	Dextran	Maltodextrin
Barley malt	Dextrose	Molasses
Beet sugar	Fructose	Powdered sugar
Bottled juice and	Galactose	Soda and soft drinks
fruit concentrates	High-fructose	Sorghum
Brown sugar	corn syrup	Syrup
Candy	Honey	White sugar
Cane juice	Malt	

Processed and Fast Foods

The Center for Food Safety estimates that at least 75 percent of processed foods on supermarket shelves contain genetically modified ingredients. Processed foods are also made with sugar, salt, grains, chemicals, and many other ingredients. A good rule when eating on this plan is to shop for ingredients, not foods. With a few exceptions, if it contains a list of ingredients, it probably isn't on this plan. Processed foods come in bags, boxes, packages, cans, jars, and bottles. Some examples of processed foods include:

Canned soups, chilies, and stews	Energy bars
Chips	Fast food
Commercial condiments such as	Frozen meals
mayonnaise and ketchup	Meal replacement bars
Commercial salad dressings	and shakes

Alcohol and Caffeine

Alcohol and caffeine are drugs that may interact in different ways in the body. Therefore, it is best to avoid consuming anything containing these substances. During the first thirty-one days of the plan, it's best to eliminate alcoholic beverages altogether. Then, try to have no more than one drink per week.

Avoid caffeine in coffee, tea, and other beverages such as cola. Caffeine is highly addictive. If you are currently consuming caffeine daily, try gradually tapering off until you no longer consume any. Herbal teas are fine, as long as they do not contain any caffeine (some herbs, such as mate and guayusa, do).

Foods to Embrace

It may be difficult to wrap your head around such a long list of foods to avoid. You may be wondering exactly what you *can* eat. Fortunately, there are many healthy, delicious foods and ingredients you can combine to make tasty, satisfying meals.

During the course of the thirty-one days of this plan, you will be able to enjoy a number of healthy, appetizing, nutrient-dense, organic foods, including succulent meats, satiating fats, mouthwatering fruits, tangy fermented foods, tasty vegetables, and flavorful herbs and spices. This food plan doesn't require you to count calories, carbohydrates, fats, or anything else. You simply get to prepare and enjoy wholesome foods that you then eat until you are no longer hungry. Since you won't be restricting calories or fats, you'll find the meals uniquely satisfying, especially if you've been subsisting on low-calorie or low-fat fare.

The best foods for you are organic, seasonal, and dense with nutrients. For every calorie of food you consume, you want to pack your body with as many

IODINE: WHAT YOU NEED TO KNOW

Many people ask about iodine and Hashimoto's thyroiditis. According to functional medicine (medicine that addresses the underlying causes of disease) specialist Chris Kresser, studies show that in countries that add iodine to table salt, rates of autoimmune thyroid disease rise. This may occur as a result of consuming too much iodine. Restricting iodine controlled autoimmune thyroiditis in 78 percent of patients. However, autoimmune thyroiditis may also occur when iodine is too low; your thyroid needs some iodine.

Fortunately, Kresser notes, high iodine intake seems to correlate with Hashimoto's only in the presence of selenium deficiency. Therefore, consuming a little bit of selenium-rich foods will minimize the impact of too much iodine on the thyroid. This amounts to eating a selenium-rich Brazil nut every other day. Before you eliminate or supplement iodine or supplement selenium, talk with your endocrinologist.

vitamins and minerals as humanly possible. The recipes in part 3 are designed to do just that.

Since you want to reduce the toxic load on your system over the next thirty-one days, seek out the most chemical-free versions of foods you can afford. That means consuming organic produce and organic, pastured meats and eggs. Select wild-caught (not farmed) seafood and organically grown herbs and vegetables.

Organic Fruits and Vegetables

For the most flavorful and nutritious foods, seek out produce that is in season. Check out your local farmers' market or co-op to discover the delicious produce in season right now.

If you can't afford all organic produce, then keep in mind a list known as the Dirty Dozen Plus. These are the fruits and vegetables that the Environmental Working Group suggests you always buy organic because they contain the highest levels of pesticides. (The produce on the Dirty Dozen Plus list changes from time to time. Find the latest list here: http://www.ewg.org/foodnews/.) They currently include:

Apples	Grapes	Peaches
Bell peppers	Hot peppers	Potatoes
Celery	Kale and collard greens	Spinach
Cherry tomatoes		Strawberries
Cucumbers	Nectarines (imported)	

Fruits and vegetables are nutritional powerhouses. They are high in fiber as well as antioxidants, which can help fight inflammation and oxidation.

However, some vegetables tend to be goitrogenic, causing thyroid hormone production to slow down. While you don't need to avoid them altogether, you may wish to minimize goitrogenic foods (that is, don't eat them every day). They include:

Bok choy	Cabbage	Mustard and mustard greens
Broccoli	Cauliflower	Radishes
Brussels sprouts	Kale	Turnips

If you are sensitive, you may also wish to avoid or minimize nightshade vegetables (see page 28).

Dairy Alternatives

Sure, dairy is out, but that doesn't mean you can't have healthy, delicious substitutes. Many offer a great way to add flavor and creaminess to recipes while packing a nutritional punch. Common dairy alternatives include:

- *Unsweetened almond milk:* Almond milk is low in calories but high in calcium and vitamin E.

- *Unsweetened coconut milk:* Coconut milk contains calcium and beneficial coconut fats. It is also a decent source of fiber and potassium.

Healthy Fats

On this plan, you don't need to fear fat. Recent research has changed the way many experts look at fat. In her book *The Big Fat Surprise*, investigative journalist Nina Teicholz explains that conventional thinking about fat is incorrect and based on inadequate science. She also states that eating saturated fats in the right kind of diet (such as this one) contributes to heart health, promotes healthy weight, and decreases inflammation.

There are a number of healthy fats you can eat and enjoy that won't contribute to inflammation. Fats to enjoy include the following:

- *Animal fats, such as duck fat, lard, chicken fat (schmaltz), and beef tallow:* These fats are all very stable at high temperatures and therefore great for cooking. These fats don't contribute to inflammation. Be sure to use fats from organic, pastured animals so they are as toxin-free as possible.

- *Avocado oil:* This oil is high in vitamin B, vitamin E, and potassium. It is mostly monounsaturated and therefore unstable at high temperatures, making it a poor choice for cooking. Use it for salad dressings, mayonnaise, and other cold applications.

- *Coconut oil:* This oil is mostly saturated, so is stable at high temperatures and less likely to oxidize when you cook with it. Coconut oil also contains medium-chain triglycerides (MCTs). According to an article in the *Journal of Nutritional Science and Vitaminology*, MCTs may help increase the number of calories your body expends, which may help prevent obesity.

ESSENTIAL VITAMINS AND MINERALS

This diet allows you to consume nutrient-dense foods, which help keep your vitamin and mineral levels well balanced. Some vitamins and minerals, however, may be especially helpful to people with Hashimoto's thyroiditis.

Vitamin D: According to Chris Kresser, vitamin D has been shown to mediate autoimmune thyroid dysfunction. Vitamin D is a fat-soluble vitamin that your body produces by absorbing sunlight. Fat-soluble vitamins can build up in the body to toxic levels, so it is important to work with your doctor when you choose to supplement vitamin D.

Living in a northern climate, wearing sunscreen, and long, cloudy winters may all reduce rates of vitamin D production, leaving you deficient in this essential nutrient. While the sun is your best source of vitamin D, it is also present in certain foods, including fatty fish like salmon, cod liver oil, portobello mushrooms, eggs, and pork.

Vitamin A: The Weston A. Price Foundation, dedicated to nutrition education, notes that vitamin A may work synergistically with vitamin D to help prevent autoimmune diseases by suppressing a certain type of inflammatory cells. Vitamin A is a fat-soluble vitamin found in a number of foods, including sweet potatoes, carrots, dark leafy greens, squash, and cantaloupe.

Selenium: As previously discussed, selenium may provide thyroid-protective benefits in diets that are too high in iodine. Likewise, selenium deficiency correlates with higher rates of autoimmune hypothyroidism, according to a study published in the *Indian Journal of Endocrinology and Metabolism*. Foods high in selenium include shiitake mushrooms, Brazil nuts, oysters, sunflower seeds, beef, and lamb.

Zinc: An Oregon State University study found that zinc deficiency was linked to increased rates of inflammation and poor immune function. Eating a diet rich in zinc may help decrease the inflammation associated with Hashimoto's. Foods that contain zinc include oysters, beef, lamb, spinach, pumpkin seeds, pork, and white mushrooms.

- **Extra-virgin olive oil:** Extra-virgin olive oil contains mostly healthy monounsaturated fats, which support a good blood cholesterol profile. Don't use olive oil for cooking, because it loses flavor. Instead, use it for cold applications such as vinaigrettes.

Nuts and Seeds (for Some)

If your body does not react adversely to nuts and seeds, they can be a wonderful part of a healthy Hashimoto's diet. Again, none of the recipes on the three-day cleanse or twenty-eight-day meal plan contain nuts or seeds, but some recipes in the book do contain them for those who can enjoy them safely after the elimination phase. These foods offer healthy fats, fiber, and a number of vitamins and minerals, such as selenium, zinc, and vitamin E. If you can consume nuts and seeds, limit your intake to an ounce or two per day. Some of the most beneficial nuts and seeds include the following:

- **Almonds:** High in vitamin E and fiber, these nuts are also a good source of potassium, iron, and magnesium. Almond flour is commonly used in place of bread crumbs in Paleo cooking, as well as in a number of baked goods and desserts.

- **Chia seeds:** When mixed with water, this excellent source of fiber makes a gel that works well as a thickener. Chia seeds are high in magnesium, calcium, and potassium.

- **Coconuts:** While not technically nuts, coconuts are a healthy source of fiber that also provide potassium, magnesium, fiber, iron, and vitamin B6. Coconut flour is an excellent substitute for grain flours in a number of dishes and desserts.

- **Macadamia nuts:** As well as being a good source of heart-healthy omega-3 fatty acids, these nuts contain magnesium, potassium, and B vitamins.

- **Walnuts:** High in anti-inflammatory omega-3 fatty acids, walnuts also contain vitamin E.

Meats, Fish, Poultry, and Eggs

These healthy foods are an excellent source of protein and fat. They also contain essential nutrients, such as vitamin B12 and iron. Meats tend to be uniquely satiating, and they also help build and repair tissue. Whenever possible, choose animal proteins that are pastured (also known as grass-fed), as they tend to be higher in anti-inflammatory omega-3 fatty acids. Select organic eggs from free-range chickens, and choose wild-caught fish and seafood.

Natural Sweeteners

There is one natural sweetener you can use over the course of the next month: stevia. Stevia comes from the stevia plant and has a natural sweetness. A little stevia goes a very long way. One teaspoon of stevia is roughly equal in sweetness to one cup of sugar.

Stevia comes in liquid extract or powder. Many stevia products are highly processed and contain other ingredients as well. Be sure to get a product that is 100 percent stevia and nothing else.

While you may find a number of natural sweeteners that are touted to fit the Paleo lifestyle, most are still sugar. For example, maple syrup, honey, and agave are all still sugar, containing mostly fructose. None of the recipes in this book contain any of the fructose-based sweeteners listed earlier in this chapter. Avoid them for at least the thirty-one days of this diet, and then you can include them in small amounts very occasionally in your diet.

PART

2

THE ACTION PLAN

CHAPTER THREE

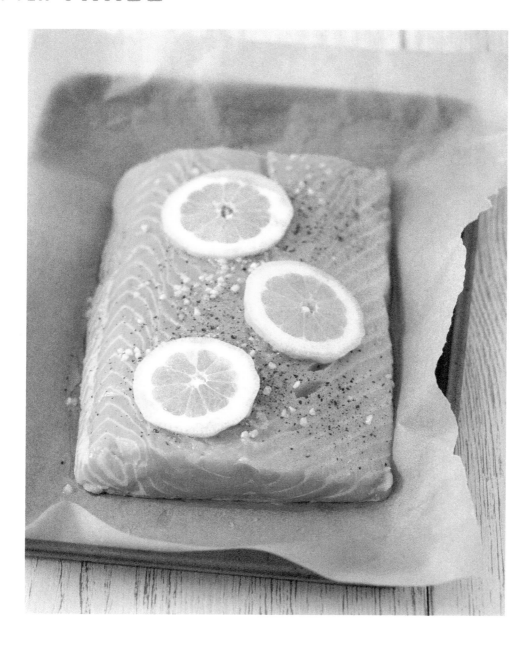

ACTION PLAN: THE ELIMINATION PHASE

In this chapter, you'll find several tools to help you make the changes necessary to improve your quality of life by changing your diet. In the first phase, you will do a three-day cleanse that helps you jump right into the changes in your diet. During the first three days, you will eliminate all the foods that may be contributing to your symptoms. The recipes will be delicious, quick, and easy, requiring thirty minutes or less of cooking. This phase of the plan will help you find the motivation to continue, and you may even notice a difference in your symptoms during the initial cleanse.

Next, you'll enter the twenty-eight-day elimination phase. During this phase, you will continue to prepare meals for yourself that eliminate the most common autoimmune symptom triggers. While some meals may require a little more time to make (and most won't!), you can make many of them ahead of time and refrigerate or freeze them.

This chapter includes meal plans and shopping lists for both phases, making it easy for you to get exactly what you need for success.

During the three-day cleanse and the twenty-eight-day elimination phase, it is important to follow the meal plans as outlined. These are the most restrictive phases of the plan, eliminating any foods that may be contributing to your Hashimoto's symptoms. In chapter 4, you will learn how to customize the diet by reintroducing some of the foods you have eliminated during your first month.

Track Your Symptoms

Before you start this meal plan for Hashimoto's, take a full inventory of your state of health. Start recording your symptoms, reactions, and emotions at least two weeks before you start the diet so you'll have a real sense of what your baseline is. If you've just purchased this book and want to start the diet right away, try to list your symptoms for at least a couple of days before beginning. This information will be your point of reference for changes that occur during the course of the diet.

Once you begin the diet, you should absolutely track your symptoms. Here are two tables that you can print (or download—see callistomediabooks.com/hashimotos) and use over the course of the next month.

Symptom Tracker / 3-Day Cleanse

		DAY 1	DAY 2	DAY 3
MORNING	Foods			
	Symptoms			
AFTERNOON	Foods			
	Symptoms			
EVENING	Foods			
	Symptoms			

Symptom Tracker / Weekly Meal Plan

		DAY 1	DAY 2	DAY 3	DAY 4	DAY 5	DAY 6	DAY 7
MORNING	Foods							
	Symptoms							
AFTERNOON	Foods							
	Symptoms							
EVENING	Foods							
	Symptoms							

If you follow the monthly plan and feel little to no improvement, it can be beneficial to discuss the situation with your doctor or another medical professional you trust to pinpoint what might be stalling your progress. You might need supplements or tests to determine the best ways to modify your approach.

It is also valuable to look very closely at how well you are complying with the food limits and to assess what's happening in your life. Here are some questions to ask yourself if you are not seeing improvements in your symptoms.

- Am I following the diet strictly?
- Am I eating a wide enough variety of thyroid and gut-health-promoting ingredients?
- Am I drinking enough water—at least eight glasses a day—and not with my meals? (Drinking water during meals dilutes the enzymes in your mouth and alters the pH in your saliva, which makes it more difficult to digest carbohydrates, starches, and sugars.)
- Am I getting eight to ten hours of sleep a night?
- Am I managing my stress?
- Do I get moderate exercise regularly?
- Are my blood sugar levels in a healthy range?

The first few days of the elimination plan—the three-day cleanse—will be difficult, even if you are enthusiastic about changing your diet. Make sure you go shopping for everything you need (pantry and shopping lists follow). The recipes for the first few days are relatively quick to make, so you can ease into this restrictive diet. You'll see suggestions for three meals a day, plus snacks. It is important that you don't skip meals—or snacks. You need to start flooding your body with nutrient-dense foods right away to help your gut heal.

The Hashimoto's diet offered here is not meant to replace any prescriptions or supplements your doctor has recommended for your autoimmune disease, although one of the goals of this healing diet might be to live your life with less medication, or even medication-free. Make sure you discuss your diet plan with your doctor before starting, because your medication might have to be adjusted.

STOCK YOUR PANTRY

The best way to begin is by creating an environment for success in your home. That's why it's important to remove or isolate foods that will no longer serve your needs (such as potato chips, bread, and processed foods), and instead stock your pantry with the foods that will bring you success. Stock your pantry with the following:

Dried Herbs and Spices

Allspice, ground
Bay leaves
Black pepper
Cinnamon, ground
Coriander
Cumin, ground
Curry powder
Fennel seed, ground
Garlic powder
Ginger, ground
Nutmeg, ground
Onion powder
Oregano
Rosemary
Sage
Sea salt
Thyme

Gluten-Free Flours

Almond meal flour
Arrowroot powder
Coconut flour
Tapioca flour

Canned and Jarred Foods

Beef broth, low-sodium
Chicken broth, low-sodium
Coconut milk, full-fat
Vegetable broth

Oil, Vinegar, and Condiments

Aminos, coconut
Animal fat (lard, chicken fat, duck fat, or tallow)
Mustard, Dijon
Oil, avocado
Oil, coconut
Oil, extra-virgin olive
Vinegar, apple cider
Vinegar, balsamic
Vinegar, red wine
Vinegar, rice wine

Non-Dairy Milk

Almond milk, unsweetened
Coconut milk, unsweetened

Sweeteners

Stevia, pure

Other Items

Baking powder
Baking soda
Vanilla extract

Gather the Tools for Success

The only way this food plan will work for you is if you follow it. I know first-hand that it requires a major lifestyle change, which can feel daunting. That's why creating an environment for success is essential to adapting to this way of eating. The effort is entirely worth it in the improved quality of life you can experience.

While you don't need a whole lot of kitchen gadgets, those listed here will help significantly in meal preparation, saving you time and energy.

Slow Cooker

If there's one tool I recommend above all others, it's a slow cooker. I actually have three that accommodate different volumes of food, because I feel they are so important in saving time and making healthy meals for my family.

Several of the recipes in this book call for a slow cooker. If you don't have one, I recommend you find a simple slow cooker that holds at least six quarts and has three settings: low, high, and keep warm. Choosing a large-capacity slow cooker enables you to make all the recipes in this book in their full amounts, and it gives you the option of making double batches so you can have leftovers, which means you can cook once and eat twice (or more!).

Food Processor

My food processor has saved me countless hours in the kitchen. While you can chop and mix by hand, a food processor can complete these types of tasks in a fraction of the time, making it the perfect tool for a busy cook.

Choose a large-capacity food processor with a chopping blade and a grater attachment.

Really Good Knife

An excellent knife is the one tool that is indispensable. The recipes in part 3 call for you to spend a lot of time chopping veggies and meat, and a good knife makes the process safer and easier. If you're only going to get one knife, make it a chef's knife, which has a long, curved blade that makes chopping easy. The best chef's knife I have ever purchased is under $50: the Victorinox Fibrox eight-inch chef's knife. If you don't have one, make sure to also get a simple knife sharpener to maintain your knife's edge.

Spiralizer

While this tool isn't essential to success, a spiralizer is still pretty great to have. It enables you to turn zucchini into noodles at the turn of a crank. I love my Paderno World Cuisine spiralizer. I use it to make zucchini noodles and the most delicious sweet potato straws. For me, it was well worth the price, which is under $50.

TIME-SAVING STRATEGIES

When you think about cooking three meals a day every day of the week, it can feel overwhelming. Even if you love to cook, spending time in the kitchen several times a day can take a huge chunk out of your free time.

One of the questions people frequently ask me is how I can find the time to cook three meals a day, every day. I have a secret: I don't. I've developed some strategies that help me keep my time in the kitchen to a minimum, so I can spend it with my family instead.

Cook once; eat twice. I make big batches of food. That way, my family can get two meals out of one cooking session. For me, it's a great way to minimize the time I spend in the kitchen.

Cook ahead. Whenever possible, I cook recipes on the weekend for use during the week. I make two big batches of broth in my slow cooker each week, and I freeze it in smaller containers. Then I just thaw what I need.

I also cook casseroles and soups ahead of time and freeze them in single servings. That way, if we don't feel like cooking dinner, or if we need to grab a fast lunch or breakfast, we can pull a single-serving container from the freezer and heat it up in our microwave.

Freeze leftovers. In the same vein, I never throw out leftovers. I always freeze them, carefully labeled, giving us more options for fast meals and snacks.

Create some simple options for meals and snacks. I always keep a carton of hardboiled eggs in my refrigerator, because they make great breakfasts or lunches. We also keep healthy snacks like nuts and seeds on hand so we can grab a quick bite on the go. You can also make up a double batch of Banana Muffins (page 80) or Pumpkin Waffles (page 82) and freeze them in individual zipper bags to grab on the go.

Make leftovers into lunches. We do this at my house—a lot. Sometimes, we even make leftovers into breakfasts.

THE THREE-DAY CLEANSE

This is the intensive start to your diet. It is designed to allow you to hit the ground running. I recommend starting on a Friday so that you are following the initial phase over the weekend. This gives you time to shop and prepare the foods for your cleanse, as well as to prepare foods ahead of time for the week to come. The recipes for the three-day cleanse and the twenty-eight-day elimination phase are found in part 3 of this book. You'll notice that the meal plans don't include dessert, even though there are dessert recipes in the book. Since we're trying to help eliminate your sweet tooth so sugar is no longer an issue, I recommend keeping desserts to a minimum (once or twice a week at most).

Meal Plan

Follow the meal plan exactly, adding in two snacks per day from the snack list.

Friday

Breakfast: Mixed Berry-Banana Smoothie

Lunch: Spinach and Shrimp Salad with Raspberry Vinaigrette

Dinner: Chicken Soup with Zucchini "Noodles"

Saturday

Breakfast: Coconut Flour Pancakes with Blueberry Compote

Lunch: Chicken Caesar Salad

Dinner: Seared Sea Scallops with Citrus Spinach

Sunday

Breakfast: Smoked Salmon Lettuce Wraps

Lunch: Egg Salad in Butter Lettuce Cups

Dinner: Turkey Piccata with Lemon Zucchini

Suggested Snacks

12 baby carrots

4 ounces deli roast beef (gluten-free)

1 sliced apple

½ sliced avocado

12 strawberries

8 ounces plain coconut milk yogurt with ¼ cup blueberries

Shopping List

Fruits and Vegetables

Apples (2)

Avocado (1)

Banana (1)

Blueberries (3 pints)

Carrots (4)

Carrots, baby (1 pound)

Celery (4 stalks)

Garlic (1 head)

Lemons (5)

Lettuce, butter (1 head)

Lettuce, romaine (2 heads)

Onions (2)

Orange (1)

Raspberries (1 pint)

Scallions (1 bunch)

Shallot (1)

Spinach, baby (3, 9-ounce packages)

Strawberries (2 pints)

Zucchini (2 medium)

Dairy Alternatives

Coconut milk, unsweetened

Coconut milk yogurt, plain

Fresh Herbs and Spices

Basil (1 bunch)

Chives (1 bunch)

Thyme (1 bunch)

Fish and Seafood

Salmon, smoked (8 ounces)

Scallops, sea (1 pound)

Shrimp, bay (1 pound)

Meat and Poultry

Chicken backs or wings, for broth
(3 pounds)

Chicken, rotisserie-cooked (1)

Chicken thighs, boneless, skinless
(16 ounces)

Roast beef, deli-sliced, gluten-free
(8 ounces)

Turkey breast, boneless, skinless
(1 pound)

Other

Capers (1 jar)

Eggs (2 dozen)

THE
3-DAY
CLEANSE

THE TWENTY-EIGHT-DAY MEAL PLAN

In the twenty-eight-day meal plan, you'll continue to eliminate the foods discussed in earlier chapters. While the meal plans list breakfast, lunch, and dinner, you may also include snacks and desserts. The snack and dessert recipes in part 3 are not factored into the shopping lists. Therefore, you'll need to plan for your snacks during the week and add the ingredients to the shopping list before you head to the grocery store.

You'll find the recipes for this meal plan in part 3. To save time, many of the recipes use a slow cooker. Others are easy to make ahead, so you can prepare foods on the weekend for the coming week. If you decide not to make a particular recipe, be sure to substitute another recipe from this cookbook in its place and adjust your shopping list accordingly.

Week 1 Meal Plan

Monday

Breakfast: Sausage and Egg Breakfast Casserole

Lunch: Mushroom, Fennel, and Italian Sausage Soup

Dinner: Steamer Clams in Lemon-Fennel Broth

Tuesday

Breakfast: Coconut Flour Porridge with Dried Fruit

Lunch: Rotisserie Chicken, Apple and Ginger Slaw

Dinner: Bacon-Wrapped Rosemary Chicken Legs with Caramelized Onion Green Beans

Wednesday

Breakfast: Fruit and Coconut Yogurt Parfait

Lunch: Leftover Bacon-Wrapped Rosemary Chicken Legs with Caramelized Onion Green Beans

Dinner: Slow Cooker Country-Style Spare Ribs with Apples and Fennel

Thursday

Breakfast: Sausage and Egg Breakfast Casserole

Lunch: Leftover Slow Cooker Country-Style Spare Ribs with Apples and Fennel

Dinner: Cod with Peach Salsa and Coconut Cauliflower "Rice"

Friday

Breakfast: Mixed Berry-Banana Smoothie

Lunch: Greek Salad with Shrimp

Dinner: Coconut Shrimp Chowder

Saturday

Breakfast: Banana Muffins

Lunch: Asparagus Crustless Quiche

Dinner: Greek-Style Lamb Burgers with Red Onion Quick Pickle, Garlic Mayonnaise, and Cucumber Salad

Sunday

Breakfast: Veggie Scramble and Banana Muffin

Lunch: Leftover Asparagus Crustless Quiche

Dinner: Baked Lemon-Dill Salmon with Celeriac Purée

Suggested Snacks

1 banana

2 celery stalks

8 ounces coconut milk yogurt and 1/2 cup sliced strawberries

2 hardboiled eggs

1/2 cup Plantain Chips

2 Refrigerator Dill Pickles

1/2 cup Zucchini "Hummus" with Carrot Sticks

Week 1 Shopping List

Fruits and Vegetables

Apples (6)

Apples, dried (4 ounces)

Arugula (1, 9-ounce bunch)

Asparagus (1 bunch)

Bananas (4)

Blueberries (1 pint)

Cantaloupe (1/2)

Carrots (8)

Cauliflower (1 head)

Celery root (celeriac) (2 bulbs)

Celery stalks (2)

Cucumbers (2)

Fennel (2 bulbs)

Garlic (4 heads)

Ginger, fresh (1 knob)

Green beans (8 ounces)

Kiwi (1)

Lemons (6)

Limes (3)

Mushrooms, button (4 ounces)

Mushrooms, cremini (8 ounces)

Onions, red (5)

Onions, yellow (10)

Peaches (3)

Radishes (8)

Raisins (4 ounces)

Raspberries (1 pint)

Spinach, baby (1, 9-ounce package)

Strawberries (1 pint)

Sweet potato (1)

Zucchini (1)

Dairy Alternatives

Coconut milk, unsweetened

Coconut milk yogurt, plain (8 ounces)

Fresh Herbs and Spices

Basil (1 bunch)

Cilantro (1 bunch)

Dill (1 bunch)

Oregano (1 bunch)

Parsley, Italian (1 bunch)

Rosemary (1 bunch)

Tarragon (1 bunch)

Thyme (1 bunch)

Fish and Seafood

Clams, steamer (2 pounds)

Cod (4 fillets totaling 16 ounces)

Salmon (4 fillets totaling 16 ounces)

Shrimp, bay (1 pound)

Shrimp, medium (1 pound)

Meat and Poultry

Bacon, thin-cut (1 pound)

Chicken, backs, wings, carcass
(for broth) (3 pounds)

Chicken, drumsticks (8)

Chicken, rotisserie-cooked (1)

Lamb, ground (1 pound)

Pork, country-style spare ribs
(2 pounds)

Pork, ground (2 pounds)

Other

Coconut milk, canned, full-fat (1)

Eggs (3 dozen)

Olives, Kalamata (2 ounces)

Week 2 Meal Plan

Monday

Breakfast: Banana Muffin and Hardboiled Egg

Lunch: Shrimp Salad with Avocado

Dinner: Slow Cooker Beef Stew

Tuesday

Breakfast: Baked Eggs and Avocados

Lunch: Leftover Slow Cooker Beef Stew

Dinner: Ground Beef and Vegetable Soup

Wednesday

Breakfast: Smoked Salmon Lettuce Wraps

Lunch: Leftover Ground Beef and Vegetable Soup

Dinner: Pumpkin Coconut Soup

Thursday

Breakfast: Banana Muffin and Hardboiled Egg

Lunch: Rotisserie Chicken with Jicama, Zucchini, and Avocado Slaw

Dinner: Shrimp Scampi with Zucchini Noodles

Friday

Breakfast: Fruit and Coconut Yogurt Parfait

Lunch: Spinach Salad with Warm Bacon Vinaigrette

Dinner: Stuffed Pork Tenderloin with Roasted Root Vegetables

Saturday

Breakfast: Pumpkin Waffles with Apple-Pear Sauce

Lunch: Leftover Rotisserie Chicken with Jicama, Zucchini, and Avocado Slaw

Dinner: Halibut with Blackberry Sauce and Asparagus

Sunday

Breakfast: Fried Eggs with Bacon and Sweet Potato Hash Browns

Lunch: Egg Salad in Butter Lettuce Cups

Dinner: Tri-Tip Roast Chimichurri with Daikon Radish Fries

Suggested Snacks

1 cup cantaloupe balls

Leftover Banana Muffin

½ avocado

¼ cup Guacamole with Jicama

2 Avocado Deviled Eggs

4 Salmon Salads with Cucumber Rounds

THE 28-DAY MEAL PLAN: WEEK 2

Week 2 Shopping List

Fruits and Vegetables

Apples (3)

Asparagus (1 pound)

Avocados (4)

Bananas (3)

Beans, green (8 ounces)

Blackberries (1 pint)

Cantaloupe (½)

Carrots (12)

Celery (5 stalks)

Celery root (celeriac) (2 bulbs)

Garlic (2 heads)

Jicama (1)

Kiwi (1)

Lemons (6)

Lettuce, butter (1 head)

Mushroom, button (8 ounces)

Mushroom, cremini (8 ounces)

Onions, yellow (4)

Parsnip (1)

Pears (3)

Radish, daikon (1 large)

Raspberries (1 pint)

Scallions (1 bunch)

Shallots (2)

Spinach, baby (2, 9-ounce packages)

Sweet potatoes (3)

Zucchini (9)

Dairy Alternatives

Coconut milk, unsweetened

Coconut yogurt, plain (8 ounces)

Fresh Herbs and Spices

Basil (1 bunch)

Chives (1 bunch)

Oregano (1 bunch)

Parsley, Italian (2 bunches)

Thyme (1 bunch)

Fish and Seafood

Halibut (4 fillets totaling 16 ounces)

Salmon, smoked (8 ounces)

Shrimp, bay (2 pounds)

Meat and Poultry

Bacon (1 pound)

Beef bones, for broth (3 pounds)

Beef, chuck roast (2 pounds)

Beef, ground (1 pound)

Beef, tri-tip roast (3 pounds)

Chicken, rotisserie-cooked (1)

Pancetta, sliced (4 ounces)

Pork, tenderloin (1 pound)

Other

Broth, vegetable (3 cups)

Eggs (3 dozen)

Pumpkin purée (2, 14-ounce cans)

Week 3 Meal Plan

Monday

Breakfast: Mixed Berry-Banana Smoothie

Lunch: Vegetable Stir-Fry with Cauliflower "Rice"

Dinner: Chicken Soup with Zucchini "Noodles"

Tuesday

Breakfast: Veggie Scramble

Lunch: Leftover Chicken Soup with Zucchini "Noodles"

Dinner: Shrimp Mojo with Mushrooms

Wednesday

Breakfast: Spinach and Herb Frittata

Lunch: Egg Salad in Butter Lettuce Cups

Dinner: Slow Cooker Horseradish Braised Beef Ribs with Cauliflower Mash

Thursday

Breakfast: Coconut Flour Porridge with Dried Fruit

Lunch: Leftover Slow Cooker Horseradish Braised Beef Ribs with Cauliflower Mash

Dinner: Coconut Shrimp Chowder

Friday

Breakfast: Baked Eggs and Avocados

Lunch: Leftover Coconut Shrimp Chowder

Dinner: Sweet Potato Curry

Saturday

Breakfast: Coconut Flour Pancakes with Blueberry Compote

Lunch: Spinach and Shrimp Salad with Raspberry Vinaigrette

Dinner: Fish Tacos

Sunday

Breakfast: Fried Eggs with Bacon and Sweet Potato Hash Browns

Lunch: Chicken Caesar Salad

Dinner: Mustard and Herb Leg of Lamb

Suggested Snacks

2 hardboiled eggs

1 cup melon balls

1 orange

2 celery stalks

½ cup Plantain Chips

2 Refrigerator Dill Pickles

1 serving Shrimp Salad with Avocado

Week 3 Shopping List

THE
28-DAY
MEAL
PLAN:
WEEK 3

Fruits and Vegetables

Apples, dried (4 ounces)

Avocados (5)

Banana (1)

Blueberries (3 pints)

Broccoli (1 bunch)

Carrots (15)

Cauliflower (2 heads)

Celery (3 stalks)

Garlic (5 heads)

Ginger, fresh (1 knob)

Horseradish (1 knob)

Lemons (3)

Lettuce, butter (1 head)

Lettuce, romaine (2 heads)

Limes (8)

Mushrooms, button (4 ounces)

Mushrooms, cremini (16 ounces)

Mushrooms, shiitake (16 ounces)

Onion, red (1)

Onions, yellow (5)

Orange (1)

Raisins (4 ounces)

Raspberries (1 pint)

Scallions (1 bunch)

Shallot (1)

Spinach, baby (2, 9-ounce packages)

Strawberries (1 pint)

Sweet potatoes (7)

Zucchini (3)

Dairy Alternatives

Coconut milk, unsweetened

Fresh Herbs and Spices

Basil (2 bunches)

Chives (2 bunches)

Cilantro (1 bunch)

Rosemary (1 bunch)

Thyme (1 bunch)

Fish and Seafood

Halibut (1 pound)

Shrimp, bay (1 pound)

Shrimp, medium (2 pounds)

Meat and Poultry

Bacon (1 pound)

Beef bones, for broth (3 pounds)

Beef, short ribs (3 pounds)

Chicken, backs, wings, or bones,
for broth (3 pounds)

Chicken, rotisserie-cooked (1)

Chicken, thighs, boneless and
skinless (1 pound)

Lamb, leg (5 pounds)

Other

Eggs (3 dozen)

Week 4 Meal Plan

Monday

Breakfast: Banana Muffins

Lunch: Leftover Mustard and Herb Leg of Lamb with Pomegranate, Blackberry, and Satsuma Salad

Dinner: Ginger Salmon with Sweet Potato Mash

Tuesday

Breakfast: Pumpkin Waffles with Apple-Pear Sauce

Lunch: Mushroom, Fennel, and Italian Sausage Soup

Dinner: Shiitake and Zucchini Hash with Poached Eggs

Wednesday

Breakfast: Sausage and Egg Breakfast Casserole

Lunch: Leftover Mustard and Herb Leg of Lamb with Apple and Ginger Slaw

Dinner: Seared Sea Scallops with Citrus Spinach

Thursday

Breakfast: Banana Muffins

Lunch: Leftover Mushroom, Fennel, and Italian Sausage Soup

Dinner: Turkey Piccata with Lemon Zucchini

Friday

Breakfast: Sausage and Egg Breakfast Casserole

Lunch: Greek Salad with Shrimp

Dinner: Ground Beef and Vegetable Soup

Saturday

Breakfast: Smoked Salmon Lettuce Wraps

Lunch: Veggie "Rice" Bowl

Dinner: Bacon-Wrapped Rosemary Chicken Legs with Caramelized Onion Green Beans

Sunday

Breakfast: Fruit and Coconut Yogurt Parfait

Lunch: Leftover Ground Beef and Vegetable Soup

Dinner: Greek-Style Lamb Burgers with Red Onion Quick Pickle, Garlic Mayonnaise, and Cucumber Salad

Suggested Snacks

4 ounces deli turkey (gluten-free)

½ cup blackberries

½ cup leftover Apple and Ginger Slaw

2 ounces smoked salmon

2 cups Kale Chips

4 Zucchini Rounds with Tapenade

½ Baked Shoestring Sweet Potato

THE
28-DAY
MEAL
PLAN:
WEEK 4

Week 4 Shopping List

Fruits and Vegetables

Apples (5)

Arugula (2, 9-ounce packages)

Bananas (2)

Beans, green (16 ounces)

Blackberries (2 pints)

Broccoli (1 bunch)

Cantaloupe (1/2)

Carrots (7)

Cauliflower (1 head)

Celery (2 stalks)

Cucumbers (4)

Fennel (1 bulb)

Garlic (2 heads)

Ginger, fresh (1 knob)

Kiwi (1)

Lemon (7)

Lettuce, butter (1 head)

Mushrooms, button (8 ounces)

Mushrooms, cremini (8 ounces)

Mushrooms, shiitake (8 ounces)

Onion, red (1)

Onions, yellow (2)

Oranges (1)

Oranges, Satsumas (8)

Pears (3)

Pomegranate seeds (1 cup)

Radishes (8)

Raspberries (1)

Scallions (1 bunch)

Shallot (1)

Spinach, baby (3, 9-ounce packages)

Sweet potatoes (2)

Zucchini (3)

Dairy Alternatives

Coconut milk, unsweetened

Coconut yogurt, plain (8 ounces)

Fresh Herbs and Spices

Chives (1 bunch)

Cilantro (1 bunch)

Oregano (1 bunch)

Parsley, Italian (2 bunches)

Rosemary (1 bunch)

Thyme (1 bunch)

Fish and Seafood

Salmon (4 fillets totaling 16 ounces)

Salmon, smoked (8 ounces)

Scallops, sea (1 pound)

Shrimp, bay (1 pound)

Meat and Poultry

Bacon (1 pound)

Beef, ground (1 pound)

Chicken, backs, wings, or bones, for broth (3 pounds)

Chicken, drumsticks (8)

Lamb, ground (1 pound)

Pork, ground (1 pound)

Pork sausage, Italian (sugar-free)
   (1 pound)

Turkey breast, boneless, skinless
   (1 pound)

Other

Asian fish sauce

Capers (2 tablespoons)

Eggs (3 dozen)

Olives, Kalamata (2 ounces)

Pumpkin purée, canned (14 ounces)

What to Expect on the Diet

If you've been eating the Standard American Diet up until now with lots of processed, fast, and restaurant foods, you will likely notice some pretty big changes when you get started. While many of the changes will be positive, you may also notice a few negative ones that often accompany any new diet, particularly one in which you are ridding yourself of addictive and/or toxic ingredients.

Positive Long-Term Changes

Some changes may come about right away. Others may take a week, two, or longer to manifest. As long as you continue to follow your healthy eating plan, you should notice that these changes last for the long term. Positive changes you might expect include:

Clearer Thinking If brain fog is part of your Hashimoto's, one of the most significant changes you may notice is in how you think. You may find your brain fog lifting, which is a wonderful thing.

Fewer Aches and Pains Feeling achy, especially in your muscles and joints, is a very common symptom for people with Hashimoto's. Changing your diet can help these symptoms start to clear.

More Energy If your Hashimoto's leaves you feeling sluggish, you may discover that your energy comes back quite quickly. I know that within a few weeks, I felt more energetic than I had in years—to the point that I almost didn't know what to do with myself.

Better Skin Whether your skin is dry or you experience lots of breakouts (both are possible with Hashimoto's, sometimes at the same time), removing all the processed foods and chemicals from your diet may help your complexion change.

Weight Loss Although this plan is not specifically a weight loss diet, in some cases, switching to a whole-foods diet, free of chemicals and processed foods, can help trigger weight loss. Since losing weight is often such a struggle with Hashimoto's, this change, if it occurs, is often a very welcome one.

Negative Short-Term Symptoms

It's hard to say exactly what you'll experience, because I don't know what type of a diet you have been eating up until now. However, if you are like most people, you've consumed the Standard American Diet, which may be high in sugar, caffeine, and chemical additives. When you abruptly cut these ingredients out of your diet, most of the changes are really positive. However, I'm not going to lie to you: You may also experience some temporary symptoms as your body fights giving up what it considers its "feel-good drugs."

Headaches Caffeine and sugar are addictive substances. When you cut them out cold turkey, you may go through a period of withdrawal. Headaches, which can be quite severe, are one symptom of withdrawal. Others include lethargy, exhaustion, and muscle aches and pains. These symptoms typically disappear after about three days.

Cravings As part of the withdrawal process, your body is going to kick up a real fuss in an attempt to get you to give it the substance to which it has grown addicted. You may notice intense cravings, particularly for sugar, bread, and other carb-filled foods. When cravings arise, feed yourself something that is on-plan. The cravings should disappear in three days to a week.

Decreased Energy You may feel a lack of energy for a few days as you withdraw from grains, sugars, and other foods. This is very temporary and should go away quite quickly. It's your body's response as it attempts to adapt to a new way of eating. In just a few days, it should begin to respond to the healthy, nutrient-dense foods you are eating.

Bowel Changes Sugar has a laxative effect on the body. As you change your diet, you may notice bowel changes—either constipation or diarrhea—as your body adapts. You will be eating a lot more fiber on this diet as well, which may also spark bowel changes. These should stop within a few days.

While these negative changes may feel discouraging, keep in mind they are short-term changes only. Within just a few days, you'll begin to feel better as your body adapts to its new way of eating.

CHAPTER FOUR

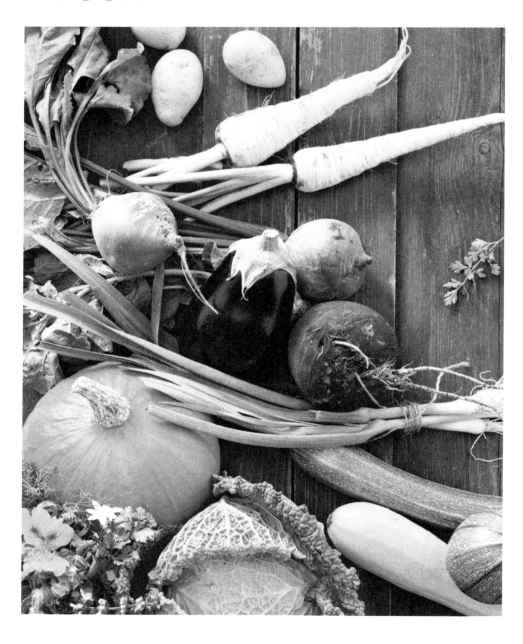

ACTION PLAN: THE REINTRODUCTION PHASE

Getting to the reintroduction phase of any plan is exciting. There's a possibility that you will be able to reincorporate into your diet some of the foods you've eliminated so far. However, some people may never be able to reincorporate certain foods. For example, I've tried to reincorporate dairy a few times. It never works out well for me. For a while, that broke my heart because I love cheese. On the other hand, I realize just how wonderful it is to feel so much better than I have for the past twenty years. For me, cheese (and the other foods I've been unable to reincorporate) simply isn't worth the reduction in quality of life.

The reincorporation phase is an important part of this plan, because it allows you to customize your diet for life. However, you can't rush the process. You need to work slowly, attempting just one food at a time, so you can learn how your body reacts to each. As you test new foods, always track your symptoms hourly, daily, and weekly so you can identify those foods that continue to give you symptoms.

As your gut heals, you may find that you can gradually add in foods later in the process, even after the reincorporation period. You can try reintroducing foods once or twice over the course of a year. However, if you continue to react to the food, chances are you'll never be able to reincorporate it.

How to Reincorporate Foods

Successfully reintroducing foods can be a huge boost to morale and make you feel excited about the prospect of again enjoying what might have been a favorite food. However, it is very important not to rush this process. The longer you allow your body to heal, the better the chance of success during the reintroductions.

You should not attempt to reintroduce any food until all your symptoms have improved considerably or subsided completely. And keep in mind that sleep, stress, and the amount of exercise you get can have a profound effect on your symptoms. You don't want to inadvertently sabotage yourself during the reintroduction process by beginning it at a time when you have a stressful work week ahead.

To the best of your ability, prepare yourself emotionally and mentally for the possibility that you might not be able to add certain foods back into your diet. But don't let this prospect scare you, because that fear response can exacerbate your symptoms. Approach the reintroduction phase as an experiment—which it is—and don't fret. Even if you can't tolerate a challenge food now, you can always try it again after six months. Food intolerances sometimes fade or change.

Reintroduce One by One

In the reintroduction phase, it can take a substantial amount of time to work through the list of eliminated foods. You have to reintroduce them one by one, so you'll know exactly how you react to that and only that food. But in the end, you will know exactly which foods can be included in your diet and which to avoid. The reintroduction process is simple, but you need to follow it strictly.

1. Pick just one challenge food, such as soy or wheat.

Adding multiple foods at once will make it difficult to determine which food might be causing any reactions you may experience.

2. Start with small amounts of the food.

Try a few bites of edamame, or start with a single whole-wheat pita. Wait for fifteen to thirty minutes to see if you have a reaction. If you have no reaction, try a greater amount of that isolated food.

3. If eating small amounts of the challenge food causes no reaction, the next day eat a normal portion of the challenge food.

Turn to chapter 14 for reintroduction recipes you can prepare at this point. If you have a reaction at any point in this process, stop eating the food and make note of it.

4. Over the next three days after eating the normal portion and having no reaction, monitor your body.

Don't eat any more of the challenge food during these three days. Reactions are not always immediate, and it can take up to three days for symptoms to manifest. Look for changes such as sleep disruption, rashes, mental fog, respiratory problems, joint pain, inflammation, exhaustion, or digestive issues. If you have any of these problems, you are intolerant and should not eat the challenge food. If you have a reaction, make sure your symptoms completely subside before trying the next challenge food. It may take a few days.

5. If after three days you have no problems, try a greater exposure to the food by eating a little every day for a week.

Sometimes reactions are more subtle than acute, and you only notice a problem when you eat the food for a week. If you have no reaction during this week-long exposure, the food is safe to add back into your diet, and you can go on to the next challenge food.

Which Foods to Reintroduce First

The foods that you will attempt to reincorporate over the next several weeks follow. Start with nightshades or nuts and seeds, and proceed with other categories in the order listed. The categories are listed from the least likely to the most likely to cause problems. And remember, reintroduce foods one by one, not a whole category at once. Sometimes one food in a group triggers symptoms, but another doesn't. For example, you may be able to eat cheddar cheese but not yogurt. Likewise, some people may be allergic to one type of legume but not another, or one type of nut but not another. Chapter 14 contains recipes that add just one reintroduced food, making it easy for you to isolate that food. This process may take several weeks, or even several months.

Nightshades

You'll notice that some of the recipes in this book contain nightshades. While those recipes aren't included in the plan, they are in the book so you can reincorporate them to see how you respond. Start with one single nightshade, such as a tomato or a hot pepper. Follow the reincorporation process described in the previous section. Consider potatoes part of the nightshade category, but give them their own reintroduction phase.

Nuts and Seeds

Some of the recipes here also contain nuts and seeds. These aren't included in meal plans but are there to provide some recipes for you when you're ready to start reincorporating this food group. Start with chia seeds or almonds.

Non-Gluten Grains

Brown rice is a great place to start with non-gluten grains. You can also try quinoa. Chapter 14 includes three recipes for reincorporating non-gluten grains.

Corn

Chapter 14 includes three corn recipes you can try, allowing you to isolate this ingredient as you attempt to determine your body's sensitivity to it.

Legumes

Follow the reintroduction recipes for legumes, or just try a small amount of your favorite beans or lentils to start.

Soy

Chapter 14 has three soy recipes for you to try. You could also start with a few pieces of edamame or a teaspoon of gluten-free soy sauce instead.

Dairy

Start with a simple dairy product like milk before moving on to a hard cheese. Chapter 14 includes three dairy recipes that isolate dairy products.

Gluten

Incorporate gluten last, since so many gluten-containing foods also contain other ingredients that have been eliminated. You'll find three gluten recipes in chapter 14.

Foods You Won't Reintroduce

Some foods are best avoided because they promote inflammation in your body. While it may have been difficult to give up these foods, it's best to avoid them altogether, or save them for very occasional indulgences.

Artificial flavors and colors	Hydrogenated oils (shortening)	Processed foods
Artificial sweeteners	Industrial seed oils	Soda
Caffeine	Preservatives	Sugar

Track Your Symptoms (Again)

During the reintroduction phase, it is important to track what you eat and your symptoms so you'll have an accurate record of what goes on in your body when you eat certain foods and how you react to them. Write everything down, both positive and negative, to get a clear idea about how foods affect your body. Keep track of other aspects of your life, too, so that a big, stressful project at work doesn't cause you to discount a challenge food.

Things to track include:

- The challenge food you are working on
- Sleep habits and how you feel when you wake up (rested, troubled, or fatigued)
- Energy levels
- Digestion
- Skin
- Emotions
- Pain and its locations (rated on a 0 to 10 scale)
- Any autoimmune disease symptoms and any changes to them
- Any other changes in your routine

The reintroduction symptom tracker chart is available for download at callistomediabooks.com/hashimotos.

Symptom Tracker / Weekly Food Reintroductions

		DAY 1	DAY 2	DAY 3	DAY 4	DAY 5	DAY 6	DAY 7
	Hours of Sleep the Night Before							
MORNING	Food Reintroduced							
	Symptoms							
AFTERNOON	Food Reintroduced							
	Symptoms							
EVENING	Food Reintroduced							
	Symptoms							
	End-of-Day Emotional Assessment							

Reintroduction FAQs

There's a good chance you have questions about reintroducing foods after reading all of this. Here are some common questions:

If I react to a food, should I eliminate it forever?

It depends. As you spend time on an anti-inflammatory diet such as this one, your gut will likely start to heal. As it does, and becomes less permeable, you may be able to reintroduce some foods you've reacted to during your initial reintroduction. I recommend giving yourself a good six to twelve months of gut healing before you attempt the food again. If the first reintroduction caused severe symptoms, I wouldn't try again.

Can I reintroduce alcohol?

Unfortunately, alcohol is a fairly inflammatory substance. It's best that you avoid it completely during your initial reintroduction phase. Once your body has had time for healing and you have been able to customize your plan, you may be able to have (and hopefully enjoy!) the occasional drink. If you do, watch for symptoms and avoid it if your body has a strong reaction.

What if I react to one food in a category, but not another?

You may have an individual allergy to a certain food within a category, but not others. That's why I recommend working your way slowly through several foods in a category instead of just assuming all foods in that category are fine. It's a long and laborious process, but it is absolutely worth it to make sure you're giving your body the best possible chance for total healing.

PART

3

HASHIMOTO'S
ACTION PLAN RECIPES

The recipes in the following chapters are intended to provide you with delicious foods that inspire you to follow the diet. While you may hear many people on diets say, "Food is just fuel to me now," the truth is that many cultural customs are largely built around sharing and enjoying meals. Eating foods you don't enjoy in order to stay on a "diet" is, over the long term, unsustainable. Therefore, the foods you'll find here are designed to not only stick to the dietary guidelines outlined in this book but to also be so tasty and enjoyable that you can share them with family and friends as part of a social and delicious meal.

Recipe Labels

Each recipe that follows starts with a series of labels that tell you how well the recipe will fit within your own personal dietary guidelines. If you have other food sensitivities or make dietary choices not covered in this book, these recipe labels can help you choose those that will work for your or your family's own specific needs.

The list of labels follows. We have also included labels that show which week's meal plan each recipe is listed in: Three-Day Cleanse, Week One, Week Two, Week Three, or Week Four.

Some of the recipes in part 3 are not included in the meal plans detailed in part 2. Because this is a lifelong diet, these recipes are here to provide variety as you continue with your customized version of the Hashimoto's plan. You will notice that some of the recipes contain nightshades and nuts. While these aren't allowed in the initial phases of the plan, you can use these recipes once you have determined you do not have a sensitivity to either of these food groups.

FODMAP-FREE

For many people with IBS, following a low-FODMAP diet can help ease the symptoms. FODMAPs are types of carbohydrates that may aggravate IBS. The foods labeled FODMAP-Free are compatible with a low-FODMAP diet.

NIGHTSHADE-FREE

As previously discussed, some people with an autoimmune disorder also have a sensitivity to nightshades, a group of vegetables that include chiles, peppers, white potatoes, eggplant, and tomatoes, among others. If you have a nightshade sensitivity, look for the recipes labeled Nightshade-Free.

NUT-FREE

Tree nuts are one of the most common allergens. Therefore, sometimes people with sensitive systems (such as people with autoimmune disease) may experience difficulties in consuming nuts.

VEGAN

Vegan recipes contain no animal products and are suitable for people on vegan diets.

VEGETARIAN

Vegetarian recipes may contain eggs but otherwise do not contain any animal products.

MAKE-AHEAD

Recipes with this label keep and reheat well. These are great recipes to cook on the weekend and either refrigerate or freeze to reheat during busy weeks.

QUICK AND EASY

You can prepare recipes with the Quick and Easy label in thirty minutes or less for total prep and cook time. These are great lunch and workday recipes.

CHAPTER FIVE

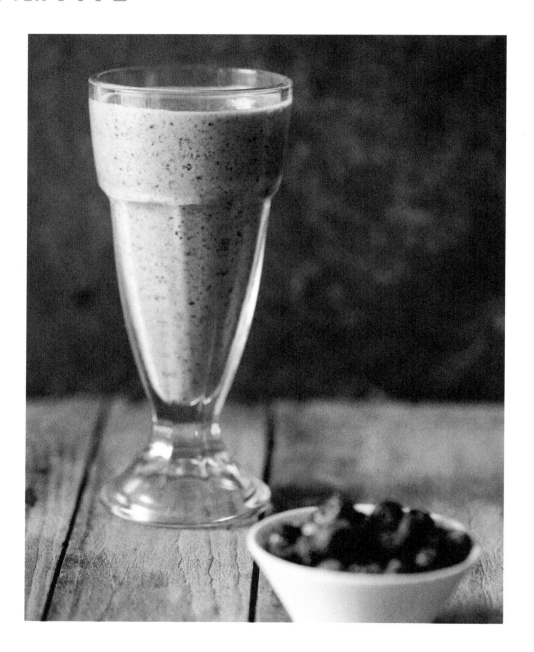

BREAKFASTS

MIXED BERRY-BANANA SMOOTHIE

Serves 2 / Prep time: 10 minutes

3-DAY CLEANSE / WEEK 1 / WEEK 3

This quick, easy breakfast is perfect for weekday mornings on the go. If you make the smoothie just for yourself, keep the rest in the refrigerator for tomorrow morning. Then, give it a quick blend in the blender to remix the ingredients.

FODMAP-FREE

NIGHTSHADE-FREE

NUT-FREE

VEGAN

QUICK & EASY

1 banana, peeled and cut into pieces
1 cup blueberries
1 cup strawberries, sliced
1 cup unsweetened coconut milk
½ teaspoon ground cinnamon

In a blender, blend the banana, blueberries, strawberries, coconut milk, and cinnamon until well combined, 1 to 2 minutes. Serve immediately.

Substitution tip: For a cold, thick smoothie, freeze the banana slices in a plastic bag before adding them to the smoothie. You can also use sugar-free frozen blueberries and strawberries in place of fresh.

PER SERVING Calories: 394; Total Fat: 29g; Saturated Fat: 25g; Cholesterol: 0mg; Carbohydrates: 37g; Fiber: 8g; Protein: 4g

FRUIT AND COCONUT YOGURT PARFAIT

Serves 2 / Prep time: 15 minutes

WEEK 1 / WEEK 2 / WEEK 4

Instead of using regular dairy yogurt, this recipe calls for coconut or almond yogurt, which you can find in the dairy aisle of your grocery store. Choose plain unsweetened yogurt for the parfaits. Fruit-on-the-bottom yogurt typically contains sugar. While this recipe calls for melon, kiwi, and raspberries, you can choose any fruit you wish.

8 ounces plain, unsweetened coconut or almond yogurt
¼ teaspoon ground nutmeg
½ teaspoon ground cinnamon
1 kiwi, peeled and sliced
1 cup raspberries
½ cup cantaloupe

1. In a small bowl, whisk together the yogurt, nutmeg, and cinnamon.
2. In two tall parfait cups, layer the yogurt mixture with the kiwi, raspberries, and cantaloupe. Serve immediately.

PER SERVING Calories: 172; Total Fat: 9g; Saturated Fat: 7g; Cholesterol: 0mg; Carbohydrates: 29g; Fiber: 14g; Protein: 2g

FODMAP-FREE

NIGHTSHADE-FREE

NUT-FREE

VEGAN

QUICK & EASY

COCONUT FLOUR PORRIDGE WITH DRIED FRUIT

Serves 2 / Prep time: 5 minutes / Cook time: 5 minutes

WEEK 1 / WEEK 3

NIGHTSHADE-
FREE

NUT-FREE

VEGAN

QUICK &
EASY

Coconut flour absorbs a lot of liquid, so it makes an excellent substitute for oatmeal on those mornings when you want a highly satisfying hot cereal. You can find coconut flour with other specialty flours in the baking aisle of the grocery store. Feel free to add more liquid to adjust the texture of the porridge just the way you like it.

1 cup unsweetened coconut milk
1 teaspoon ground cinnamon
Pinch sea salt
½ teaspoon stevia
½ cup coconut flour
½ cup dried apples
½ cup raisins

1. In a medium saucepan over medium-high heat, bring the coconut milk, cinnamon, sea salt, and stevia to a simmer.

2. Remove the pan from the heat and stir in the coconut flour, dried apples, and raisins.

3. Let sit for 1 to 2 minutes before serving.

PER SERVING Calories: 290; Total Fat: 7g; Saturated Fat: 4g; Cholesterol: 0mg; Carbohydrates: 55g; Fiber: 16g; Protein: 8g

GRAIN-FREE GRANOLA

Serves 6 / Prep time: 20 minutes / Cook time: 20 minutes

If you enjoy a morning meal of granola, this is a great substitute. Made with nuts and seeds and sweetened with dates, it offers all of the flavor and crunch of granola without the grains. Feel free to substitute your favorite nuts and seeds for any in this recipe.

○

NIGHTSHADE-
FREE

○

VEGAN

1 cup medjool dates
1 cup water
2 cups almonds
2 cups walnuts
1 cup pumpkin seeds
½ cup unsweetened coconut flakes
1 teaspoon vanilla extract
½ teaspoon sea salt
3 cups unsweetened almond milk

1. In a small bowl, combine the dates and water. Cover with plastic wrap and soak overnight.

2. Preheat the oven to 325°F.

3. Line a baking sheet with parchment paper.

4. In a food processor, pulse the almonds, walnuts, and pumpkin seeds for 10 one-second pulses. Transfer the nuts to a large bowl. Add the coconut flakes.

5. Add the soaked dates and water, vanilla, and sea salt to the food processor and blend until smooth, about 1 minute.

6. Pour the date mixture over the nuts and mix thoroughly.

7. Spread the mixture on the prepared baking sheet. Bake for about 20 minutes, stirring every 5 minutes.

8. Allow the mixture to cool thoroughly, and serve each bowl topped with ½ cup almond milk.

PER SERVING Calories: 582; Total Fat: 52g; Saturated Fat: 5g; Cholesterol: 0mg; Carbohydrates: 16g; Fiber: 8g; Protein: 23g

COCONUT FLOUR PANCAKES WITH BLUEBERRY COMPOTE

Serves 4 / Prep time: 10 minutes / Cook time: 10 minutes

3-DAY CLEANSE / WEEK 3

FODMAP-
FREE

NIGHTSHADE-
FREE

NUT-FREE

VEGETARIAN

QUICK &
EASY

Coconut flour has a relatively neutral taste that substitutes well for wheat flour in pancakes. Because coconut flour absorbs liquid so readily, don't make the batter ahead of time. Make the batter within about 10 minutes of cooking it. Then, top the pancakes with the warm blueberry compote for a classic breakfast.

FOR THE PANCAKES

½ cup coconut flour

¼ teaspoon baking soda

Pinch sea salt

½ cup unsweetened coconut milk

¼ cup coconut oil, melted, plus more for cooking

3 eggs, slightly beaten

1 teaspoon vanilla extract

FOR THE COMPOTE

2 cups blueberries (fresh or frozen)

1 teaspoon ground cinnamon

¼ cup water

½ teaspoon stevia

TO MAKE THE PANCAKES

1. In a medium-size bowl, whisk together the coconut flour, baking soda, and sea salt.

2. In a large bowl, whisk together the coconut milk, coconut oil, eggs, and vanilla.

3. Add the wet ingredients to the dry ingredients and fold together until just combined.

4. Heat a large skillet over medium-high heat. Coat the skillet with melted coconut oil.

5. Pour in the batter in ¼-cup portions and cook. When the underside of the pancake has browned, flip the pancake and continue cooking, 5 to 7 minutes total for both sides.

TO MAKE THE COMPOTE

1. In a medium saucepan, heat the blueberries, cinnamon, water, and stevia over medium-high heat. Bring to a simmer and cook until the blueberries pop and start to thicken, about 10 minutes.

2. Serve the pancakes with the compote spooned over the top.

PER SERVING Calories: 284; Total Fat: 20g; Saturated Fat: 15g; Cholesterol: 123mg; Carbohydrates: 21g; Fiber: 8g; Protein: 8g

BANANA MUFFINS

Serves 6 / Prep time: 10 minutes / Cook time: 20 minutes

WEEK 1 / WEEK 2 / WEEK 4

This recipe is a great way to use overripe bananas. In fact, use bananas with skin that has turned brown. This level of ripeness makes the bananas easier to work with and increases their natural sugars. Just don't overmix the batter—it's okay if the batter has lumps and a few streaks of flour in it.

2 bananas, very ripe, peeled and mashed

1 teaspoon stevia

4 eggs

¼ cup coconut oil, melted

½ cup coconut milk

1 teaspoon vanilla extract

½ cup coconut flour

½ cup tapioca flour

½ teaspoon ground cinnamon

½ teaspoon baking soda

½ teaspoon baking powder

¼ teaspoon sea salt

1. Preheat the oven to 375°F. Line 6 cups of a muffin tin with paper liners.

2. In a medium bowl, whisk together the mashed bananas, stevia, eggs, coconut oil, coconut milk, and vanilla.

3. In a large bowl, whisk together the coconut flour, tapioca flour, cinnamon, baking soda, baking powder, and sea salt.

4. Add the wet ingredients to the dry ingredients and fold together until just combined.

5. Bake until a toothpick inserted in the muffins comes out clean, about 20 minutes. Cool on a wire rack before serving.

PER SERVING Calories: 279; Total Fat: 19g; Saturated Fat: 5g; Cholesterol: 41mg; Carbohydrates: 72g; Fiber: 4g; Protein: 7g

FODMAP-FREE

NIGHTSHADE-FREE

NUT-FREE

VEGETARIAN

MAKE-AHEAD

QUICK & EASY

TOMATO, BACON, AND AVOCADO BREAKFAST SALAD

Serves 4 / Prep time: 10 minutes / Cook time: 5 minutes

Tomatoes, bacon, and avocados make a classic flavor combination. The sweetness of the tomatoes contrasts perfectly with the creamy avocados and smoky bacon. This recipe tastes its best when tomatoes are in season during the summer. Stop by your local farmers' market and pick out some beautiful, juicy heirloom tomatoes.

○
NUT-FREE

○
QUICK & EASY

8 slices thick-cut bacon

2 large heirloom tomatoes

1 avocado, peeled, pitted, and cut into pieces

1 cup baby arugula

Juice of ½ lemon

1. In a large sauté pan over medium-high heat, cook the bacon slices until they are crispy. Blot the bacon on a paper towel; then cut it into ¼-inch pieces. Put the bacon in a large bowl.

2. Chop the tomatoes, and add them to the bowl with the bacon.

3. Add the avocado and arugula.

4. Squeeze the lemon juice over the salad, toss to combine, and serve.

Ingredient tip: Check with your local butcher shop to find a tasty, uncured, artisanal bacon to add even more flavor to this dish.

PER SERVING Calories: 303; Total Fat: 24g; Saturated Fat: 7g; Cholesterol: 30mg; Carbohydrates: 9g; Fiber: 5g; Protein: 12g

PUMPKIN WAFFLES WITH APPLE-PEAR SAUCE

Serves 4 / Prep time: 5 minutes / Cook time: 20 minutes

WEEK 2 / WEEK 4

FODMAP-
FREE

NIGHTSHADE-
FREE

VEGETARIAN

MAKE-AHEAD

QUICK &
EASY

Top these tasty waffles with a homemade apple-pear sauce for a filling, delicious breakfast. You can eat these waffles warm, or make them ahead and eat them cold for breakfast on the go. Be sure you use unsweetened canned pumpkin and not pumpkin pie mix, which has sugar and milk in it.

½ cup pumpkin purée

¼ cup unsweetened coconut milk

2 eggs

¼ cup melted coconut oil, plus more for brushing

1 teaspoon vanilla extract

½ cup tapioca flour

¼ cup coconut flour

⅛ teaspoon baking powder

⅛ teaspoon baking soda

1 teaspoon ground cinnamon

¼ teaspoon ground nutmeg

¼ teaspoon ground allspice

Pinch sea salt

1 cup Apple-Pear Sauce (page 221)

1. Preheat a waffle iron.

2. In a medium bowl, whisk together the pumpkin, coconut milk, eggs, coconut oil, and vanilla.

3. In another medium bowl, whisk together the tapioca flour, coconut flour, baking powder, baking soda, cinnamon, nutmeg, allspice, and salt.

4. Add the wet ingredients to the dry ingredients and fold together until just combined.

5. Pour the batter in ¼-cup portions onto a greased waffle iron. Cook until the waffles are done, about 5 minutes each.

6. Serve each waffle topped with Apple-Pear Sauce.

Cooking tip: If you don't have a waffle iron, you can make these as pancakes. Scoop the mixture by scant ¼-cup portions onto a preheated nonstick griddle or pan over medium-high heat, greased with coconut oil. Cook for about 3 minutes per side, until browned.

PER SERVING Calories: 309; Total Fat: 29g; Saturated Fat: 14g; Cholesterol: 82mg; Carbohydrates: 8g; Fiber: 3g; Protein: 8g

SMOKED SALMON LETTUCE WRAPS

Serves 4 / Prep time: 5 minutes / Cook time: 8 minutes

3-DAY CLEANSE / WEEK 2 / WEEK 4

Lettuce makes the perfect substitute for tortillas in wraps. While you can use any type of lettuce, romaine and butter lettuce work best. Choose the large outer leaves, which are best for wraps. Choose a sugar-free smoked salmon, if you can. If you can't find sugar-free, choose the salmon with the fewest grams of sugar per serving (1 gram or less).

NIGHTSHADE-
FREE

NUT-FREE

QUICK &
EASY

1 tablespoon animal fat, such as lard or duck fat

6 eggs, beaten

Zest of ½ lemon

¼ teaspoon sea salt

¼ teaspoon freshly ground black pepper

8 ounces smoked salmon, cut in small pieces

2 tablespoons chopped fresh chives

4 large pieces butter lettuce leaves

1. In a nonstick sauté pan over medium-high heat, heat the fat.

2. In a small bowl, whisk together the eggs, lemon zest, salt, and pepper.

3. Scramble the eggs in the preheated pan, stirring frequently, until they are cooked through, about 4 minutes.

4. Add the salmon and chives. Cook, stirring frequently, until the salmon is warmed through, about 1 minute.

5. Wrap the egg mixture in the lettuce leaves to serve.

Substitution tip: For a FODMAP-Free version of this recipe, replace the chives with the chopped green parts from a scallion (sometimes called green onion).

PER SERVING Calories: 190; Total Fat: 12g; Saturated Fat: 4g; Cholesterol: 1mg; Carbohydrates: 1g; Fiber: 0g; Protein: 19g

VEGGIE SCRAMBLE

Serves 4 / Prep time: 10 minutes / Cook time: 10 minutes

WEEK 1 / WEEK 3

The best part of this recipe is its versatility. While it calls for specific vegetables, you can mix it up by adding any veggies you wish. Try grated carrots, sweet bell peppers (if you aren't sensitive to nightshades), or fennel in place of the other vegetables. Use this recipe as a template to make your own delicious veggie scramble.

1 tablespoon extra-virgin olive oil
½ onion, chopped
1 zucchini, chopped
4 ounces button mushrooms, sliced
8 eggs, beaten
½ teaspoon sea salt
¼ teaspoon freshly ground black pepper
2 tablespoons chopped fresh basil

NIGHTSHADE-FREE

NUT-FREE

VEGETARIAN

QUICK & EASY

1. In a nonstick sauté pan over medium-high heat, heat the olive oil.

2. Add the onion, zucchini, and mushrooms to the pan and cook, stirring occasionally, until the vegetables are soft, about 5 minutes.

3. In a medium bowl, whisk together the eggs, salt, and pepper. Add the mixture to the pan and cook, stirring frequently, until the eggs are done, about 5 minutes more.

4. Remove from the heat, stir in the basil, and serve.

Substitution tip: For a FODMAP-Free version, eliminate the mushrooms and onion. Replace the onions with the chopped green parts of three scallions, and replace the mushrooms with a FODMAP-friendly vegetable, such as spinach.

PER SERVING Calories: 176; Total Fat: 13g; Saturated Fat: 3g; Cholesterol: 327mg; Carbohydrates: 5g; Fiber: 1g; Protein: 13g

FRIED EGGS WITH BACON AND SWEET POTATO HASH BROWNS

Serves 4 / Prep time: 10 minutes / Cook time: 25 minutes

WEEK 2 / WEEK 3

FODMAP-
FREE

NIGHTSHADE-
FREE

NUT-FREE

Because this recipe takes a little longer to cook, it's a perfect weekend breakfast. Slide an over-easy fried egg onto a bed of sweet potato hash browns, and let the runny yolk serve as the "sauce." Of course, if you prefer to keep everything separate on your plate, just put the eggs off to the side. Cook up the bacon first, and use the fat to cook the hash browns for a smoky flavor.

8 slices bacon

2 sweet potatoes, peeled and shredded

1 teaspoon sea salt, divided

½ teaspoon freshly ground black pepper, divided

4 eggs

2 tablespoons chopped fresh chives (optional)

1. Preheat the oven to 200°F.

2. In a nonstick sauté pan, cook the bacon until it is crisp and the fat is rendered, about 3 minutes per side. Using tongs, remove the bacon from the pan. Blot it on paper towels, and put it on an oven-safe plate. Put the bacon in the preheated oven to keep warm.

3. Remove all but 2 tablespoons of bacon grease from the sauté pan and set it aside.

4. In the sauté pan over medium-high heat, heat the remaining 2 tablespoons bacon grease. Add the shredded potatoes. Season them with ¾ teaspoon salt and ¼ teaspoon pepper.

5. Cook without turning the hash browns until they begin to brown on one side, about 5 minutes. Flip the hash browns and continue cooking, allowing them to brown on the other side, another 5 minutes. Remove the hash browns from the pan and divide them among four plates.

6. Add 2 more tablespoons of bacon fat to the pan and return it to medium heat. When the fat is hot, crack the eggs into the pan, making sure they don't touch one another. Sprinkle them with the remaining salt and pepper.

7. Cook until the whites are opaque, about 4 minutes. Flip the eggs and turn off the heat. Leave the eggs to sit in the hot pan for 1 minute.

8. Add the reserved bacon to the plates. Put the eggs on top of the hash browns.

9. Sprinkle the eggs with the chopped chives (if using) and serve.

Ingredient tip: To shred the sweet potato, use a food processor with a shredding disc, or use a box grater.

PER SERVING Calories: 503; Total Fat: 29g; Saturated Fat: 9g; Cholesterol: 226mg; Carbohydrates: 33g; Fiber: 5g; Protein: 29g

SPINACH AND HERB FRITTATA

Serves 4 / Prep time: 10 minutes / Cook time: 15 minutes

WEEK 3

Use an ovenproof pan for this frittata. A good choice is a well-seasoned 12-inch cast iron skillet. Don't use a pan with a plastic handle because it will melt.

NIGHTSHADE-
FREE

NUT-FREE

VEGETARIAN

QUICK &
EASY

8 eggs
1 tablespoon chopped fresh thyme
1 tablespoon chopped fresh chives
Zest of 1 orange
½ teaspoon sea salt
½ teaspoon freshly ground black pepper
2 tablespoons extra-virgin olive oil
2 tablespoons minced shallots
2 cups baby spinach
3 garlic cloves, minced

1. Preheat the broiler to high.
2. In a large bowl, whisk together the eggs, thyme, chives, orange zest, sea salt, and pepper. Set aside.
3. In a large ovenproof sauté pan over medium-high heat, heat the olive oil until it shimmers. Add the shallots and cook, stirring frequently, until they are soft, about 3 minutes.
4. Add the spinach and cook, stirring frequently, until it is soft and wilted, about 2 minutes more.
5. Add the garlic and cook, stirring constantly, until the garlic is fragrant, about 30 seconds.
6. Pour the egg mixture carefully over the vegetables. Cook without stirring until the bottom sets, about 3 minutes.
7. Move the pan to the oven and set it under the broiler, cooking until the top sets, another 3 or 4 minutes.
8. Cut into wedges and serve.

PER SERVING Calories: 199; Total Fat: 16g; Saturated Fat: 4g; Cholesterol: 327mg; Carbohydrates: 3g; Fiber: 1g; Protein: 12g

BAKED EGGS AND AVOCADOS

Serves 4 / Prep time: 4 minutes / Cook time: 20 minutes

WEEK 2 / WEEK 3

This quick recipe is really easy, really fast, and really delicious. The avocado serves as the perfect vessel for the egg, so you have a self-contained meal within the avocado half. You'll need to scoop out a little bit of the avocado flesh to accommodate the egg. Rub it with lemon juice, and set it aside in an airtight container for later use in a salad or purée.

2 avocados, halved and pitted
½ lemon
4 eggs
Sea salt
Freshly ground black pepper

NIGHTSHADE-FREE

NUT-FREE

VEGETARIAN

QUICK & EASY

1. Preheat the oven to 425°F.

2. Scoop some of the flesh out of the center of each avocado half to make room for the eggs.

3. Arrange the avocado halves, cut-side up, on a baking sheet. Rub the cut side of the avocados with the lemon half.

4. Crack 1 egg into each avocado half.

5. Season with salt and pepper.

6. Bake until the eggs set, about 20 minutes.

7. Serve immediately.

PER SERVING Calories: 268; Total Fat: 24g; Saturated Fat: 6g; Cholesterol: 164mg; Carbohydrates: 9g; Fiber: 7g; Protein: 8g

SAUSAGE AND EGG BREAKFAST CASSEROLE

Serves 8 / Prep time: 10 minutes / Cook time: 30 minutes

WEEK 1 / WEEK 4

This is a great casserole to make on the weekends so that you have it on hand and ready to heat throughout the week (as the meal plan indicates). Store it in the refrigerator in a tightly sealed container, or in the freezer in individual slices. What takes just a bit of time to make is the sausage itself. If this doesn't appeal to you, you can look for store-bought sausage that is sugar-free.

FOR THE SAUSAGE

1 pound ground pork

1½ teaspoons ground sage

1 teaspoon ground fennel seed

1 teaspoon garlic powder

½ teaspoon sea salt

½ teaspoon freshly ground black pepper

FOR THE CASSEROLE

Coconut oil, for greasing

12 eggs

½ cup coconut milk

½ teaspoon sea salt

½ teaspoon freshly ground black pepper

½ teaspoon garlic powder

2 cups baby spinach leaves

½ cup Slow Cooker Caramelized Onions (page 228)

TO MAKE THE SAUSAGE

1. In a large bowl, mix the pork, sage, fennel, garlic powder, salt, and pepper until well combined.

2. In a large sauté pan over medium-high heat, cook the sausage, stirring frequently, until it is cooked through, about 5 minutes.

3. Drain the fat from the sausage, and allow it to cool slightly.

TO MAKE THE CASSEROLE

1. Preheat the oven to 400°F.

2. Grease a 9-by-13-inch baking dish with coconut oil.

3. In a large bowl, whisk together the eggs, coconut milk, salt, pepper, and garlic powder until well combined.

4. Fold in the cooled sausage, spinach, and Slow Cooker Caramelized Onions.

5. Pour the mixture into the prepared pan and bake until it is cooked through, about 30 minutes, and serve.

PER SERVING Calories: 215; Total Fat: 12g; Saturated Fat: 6g; Cholesterol: 287mg; Carbohydrates: 2g; Fiber: 1g; Protein: 24g

SPICY CHORIZO, SWEET POTATO, AND EGG CASSEROLE

Serves 8 / Prep time: 10 minutes / Cook time: 30 minutes

This casserole starts your day off with a kick. The homemade chorizo adds a wonderful, spicy flavor for people who like their mornings to be zippy. If you need to cool it down a bit, serve the casserole with slices of avocado on the side.

NUT-FREE

MAKE-AHEAD

FOR THE CHORIZO

1 pound ground pork

¾ teaspoon ground cumin

¼ teaspoon ground cinnamon

½ teaspoon garlic powder

½ teaspoon dried oregano

¼ teaspoon ground coriander

2 tablespoons chili powder

½ teaspoon chipotle powder

½ teaspoon sea salt

½ teaspoon freshly ground black pepper

FOR THE CASSEROLE

Coconut oil, for greasing

12 eggs

½ cup almond milk

½ teaspoon sea salt

½ teaspoon freshly ground black pepper

1 sweet potato, peeled and shredded

TO MAKE THE CHORIZO

1. In a large bowl, mix the pork, cumin, cinnamon, garlic powder, oregano, coriander, chili powder, chipotle powder, salt, and pepper.

2. In a large sauté pan over medium-high heat, cook the chorizo, stirring frequently, until it is cooked through, about 5 minutes.

3. Drain the fat from the chorizo, and allow it to cool slightly.

TO MAKE THE CASSEROLE

1. Preheat the oven to 400°F.

2. Grease a 9-by-13-inch baking dish with coconut oil.

3. In a large bowl, whisk together the eggs, almond milk, salt, and pepper until well combined.

4. Fold in the cooled chorizo and the sweet potato.

5. Pour the mixture into the prepared pan and bake until it is cooked through, about 30 minutes, and serve.

PER SERVING Calories: 266; Total Fat: 21g; Saturated Fat: 9g; Cholesterol: 197mg; Carbohydrates: 4g; Fiber: 1g; Protein: 15g

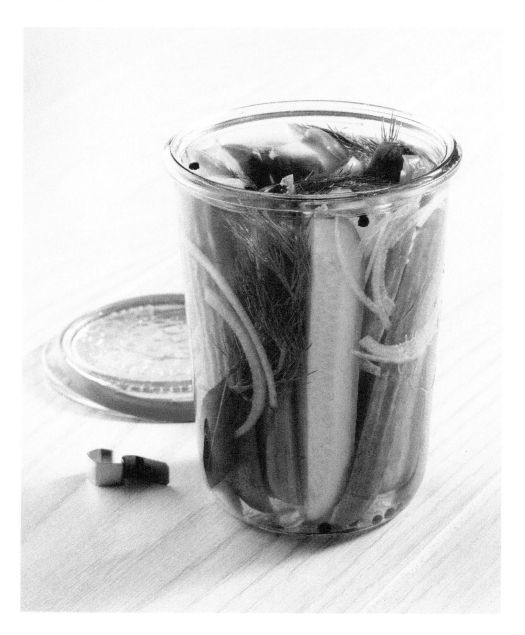

SNACKS

COCONUT CREAM with STRAWBERRIES

Serves 4 / Prep time: 10 minutes / Cook time: 10 minutes

This snack is so simple, yet so satisfying. With pillowy coconut cream and sweet berries, it offers you a little something sweet. The coconut milk makes it fatty enough, however, that the dish will satisfy you until your next meal. This recipe is best when local strawberries are in season in late June and early July. You can also substitute other seasonal berries.

½ cup unsweetened coconut flakes
4 cups fresh strawberries, sliced
1 cup Coconut Cream (page 214)

1. Preheat the oven to 325°F.

2. Line a baking sheet with parchment paper.

3. Spread the coconut flakes in a single layer on the prepared baking sheet. Bake until they brown, about 10 minutes. Allow them to cool completely.

4. Slice the strawberries into four bowls, and spoon the Coconut Cream over the top of each.

5. Sprinkle the toasted coconut on top of the coconut cream and serve.

PER SERVING Calories: 219; Total Fat: 18g; Saturated Fat: 16g; Cholesterol: 0mg; Carbohydrates: 16g; Fiber: 5g; Protein: 3g

FODMAP-FREE

NIGHTSHADE-FREE

NUT-FREE

VEGAN

QUICK & EASY

APPLES WITH ALMOND BUTTER DIP

Serves 6 / Prep time: 10 minutes

Make this dip ahead of time, and take it with you in a tightly sealed container for a quick, high-energy snack. You can use this almond butter dip with any fruits or vegetables you wish, such as celery, berries, or pears.

1½ cups almond butter
½ cup almond milk
1 teaspoon ground cinnamon
1 packet stevia
Pinch sea salt
3 apples, cored and sliced

1. In the bowl of a food processor, process the almond butter, almond milk, cinnamon, stevia, and sea salt until blended, about 30 seconds.
2. Scrape the mixture into a bowl, and serve as a dip for the apple slices.

Ingredient tip: If you plan to slice the apples and take them with you, toss them with the juice of a lemon to keep them from turning brown. Then put the apples in a tightly sealed container.

PER SERVING Calories: 491; Total Fat: 40g; Saturated Fat: 8g; Cholesterol: 0mg; Carbohydrates: 25g; Fiber: 5g; Protein: 14g

NIGHTSHADE-FREE

VEGAN

MAKE-AHEAD

QUICK & EASY

FRUIT SALAD WITH COCONUT CREAM

Serves 6 / Prep time: 10 minutes / Cook time: 10 minutes

If you're a fan of ambrosia salad, this is a worthy substitute. It uses healthy coconut cream in place of chemical-laden whipped topping. It also uses fresh fruit in place of the high-sugar, syrupy canned fruit in the classic recipe.

NIGHTSHADE-
FREE

NUT-FREE

VEGAN

MAKE-AHEAD

QUICK &
EASY

1 cup unsweetened coconut flakes

1 banana, sliced

2 cups green grapes, halved

3 satsuma oranges, peeled and sectioned

2 apples, peeled, cored, and chopped

1 cup Coconut Cream (page 214)

1. Preheat the oven to 325°F.

2. Line a baking sheet with parchment paper.

3. Spread the coconut flakes in a single layer on the prepared baking sheet. Bake until they are browned, about 10 minutes. Allow them to cool.

4. In a large bowl, stir together the cooled coconut flakes, banana, grapes, orange sections, and apples.

5. Add the coconut cream, and stir until well combined. Serve chilled.

PER SERVING Calories: 223; Total Fat: 14g; Saturated Fat: 13g; Cholesterol: 0mg; Carbohydrates: 25g; Fiber: 19g; Protein: 2g

SPICED PECANS

Serves 4 / Prep time: 10 minutes / Cook time: 10 minutes

These toasty, spicy nuts make a filling snack, so they are great when you have a while to go before your next meal. They also travel well and keep for a few weeks in a tightly sealed container. Feel free to substitute some other type of nut if you prefer.

1 cup pecan halves
1 packet stevia
¼ teaspoon ground cinnamon
¼ teaspoon ground cloves
¼ teaspoon ground nutmeg
¼ teaspoon sea salt
2 tablespoons melted coconut oil

1. In a large sauté pan over medium-high heat, toast the pecans, stirring often, until they smell toasty, about 4 minutes.

2. In a small bowl, mix the stevia, cinnamon, cloves, nutmeg, and salt.

3. In a medium bowl, toss the pecan halves with the melted coconut oil and the spice mixture.

4. Allow to cool before serving.

Ingredient tip: If you aren't sensitive to nightshades and want a spicier nut, add ⅛ teaspoon of cayenne pepper to the seasoning blend.

PER SERVING Calories: 304; Total Fat: 32g; Saturated Fat: 8g; Cholesterol: 0mg; Carbohydrates: 5g; Fiber: 4g; Protein: 4g

NIGHTSHADE-FREE

VEGAN

MAKE-AHEAD

QUICK & EASY

KALE CHIPS

Serves 4 / Prep time: 10 minutes / Cook time: 20 minutes

Kale is a nutritious food that is high in vitamins A and C. While kale is considered a goitrogen, as long as you don't eat it every day, it shouldn't affect you that much. These chips will store well in a tightly sealed container for up to a week, so they are a good make-ahead snack.

NIGHTSHADE-FREE

NUT-FREE

VEGAN

MAKE-AHEAD

1 bunch kale, washed and dried
2 tablespoons coconut oil, melted
½ teaspoon sea salt
½ teaspoon freshly ground black pepper
½ teaspoon garlic powder
½ teaspoon onion powder

1. Preheat the oven to 275°F.
2. Line a baking sheet with parchment paper.
3. Remove the ribs from the kale, and tear it into bite-size pieces.
4. In a large bowl, toss the kale with the coconut oil, salt, pepper, garlic powder, and onion powder.
5. Spread the kale on the baking sheet in a single layer.
6. Bake the kale, stirring and turning it occasionally, until it is crisp, about 20 minutes.
7. Cool and serve.

Cooking tip: It is extremely important to use dry kale. Wash the kale thoroughly in running water. Then blot it with paper towels or use a salad spinner to dry it thoroughly.

PER SERVING Calories: 86; Total Fat: 7g; Saturated Fat: 6g; Cholesterol: 0mg; Carbohydrates: 6g; Fiber: 1g; Protein: 2g

PLANTAIN CHIPS

Serves 4 / Prep time: 10 minutes / Cook time: 10 minutes

Plantain is a starchy variety of banana that is similar in taste to potatoes. Find it in the produce section of the grocery store near the bananas. Plantain chips are a traditional snack in Puerto Rico, where they are called tostones.

½ cup coconut oil
2 plantains, peeled and sliced
Cold water, for dipping
½ teaspoon sea salt

1. In a large sauté pan over medium-high heat, heat the coconut oil until it is shimmering hot.

2. Add the plantains and fry them in the oil, 4 minutes per side.

3. Remove the plantains from the oil, and flatten each one with a fork.

4. Dip the plantains in a bowl of cold water, and return them to the hot oil. Fry them for 1 minute per side.

5. Blot on a paper towel, season with salt, and serve warm.

PER SERVING Calories: 168; Total Fat: 7g; Saturated Fat: 6g; Cholesterol: 0mg; Carbohydrates: 29g; Fiber: 2g; Protein: 2g

NIGHTSHADE-FREE

NUT-FREE

VEGAN

MAKE-AHEAD

QUICK & EASY

BAKED SHOESTRING SWEET POTATOES

Serves 2 / Prep time: 10 minutes / Cook time: 20 minutes

These sweet potatoes make a delicious substitute for French fries. Cutting them very thin leaves them crispy on the outside and tender on the inside. You can cut the potatoes by hand, or use a mandoline slicer. You can also use a special kitchen tool called a spiralizer, which many Paleo cooks use to turn zucchini into pasta and sweet potatoes into shoestrings.

1 sweet potato, peeled and cut into very thin shoestrings
2 tablespoons animal fat, such as duck fat or lard
Sea salt to taste

FODMAP-
FREE

NIGHTSHADE-
FREE

NUT-FREE

QUICK &
EASY

1. Preheat the oven to 400°F.

2. Line a baking sheet with parchment paper.

3. In a large bowl, toss the sweet potato strips with the fat and the salt.

4. Place the potatoes in a single layer on the baking sheet. Bake until they are crisp and golden, about 20 minutes, and serve.

Ingredient tip: Many stores carry a variety of sweet potatoes. These shoestrings work particularly well with the white-fleshed sweet potatoes.

PER SERVING Calories: 167; Total Fat: 13g; Saturated Fat: 5g; Cholesterol: 12mg; Carbohydrates: 12g; Fiber: 2g; Protein: 1g

REFRIGERATOR DILL PICKLES

Serves 8 / Prep time: 15 minutes / Cook time: 5 minutes

These dill pickles will keep in your refrigerator for about a month. Make them in wide-mouthed Mason jars so you can easily add all the ingredients and pour in the brine. It will take the pickles about a week to fully cure in the brine.

2 cups white wine vinegar

2 cups water

¼ cup pickling salt

1½ pounds pickling cucumbers, quartered lengthwise

12 garlic cloves, crushed

¼ onion, thinly sliced

6 sprigs dill

½ tablespoon cracked black peppercorns

NUT-FREE

VEGAN

MAKE-AHEAD

QUICK & EASY

1. In a large saucepan, bring the vinegar, water, and salt to a boil. Boil until the salt dissolves, then remove from the heat.

2. While the brine cooks, distribute the cucumbers, garlic cloves, onion, dill, and peppercorns evenly between 2 one-quart Mason jars.

3. Pour the hot brine over the cucumbers in the Mason jars. Allow them to cool to room temperature.

4. Seal the jars with the lids and rings, and refrigerate for about a week before eating.

Substitution tip: Pickling salt keeps pickles from discoloring. However, if you wish, you can use sea salt. If you use sea salt, only use 2 tablespoons in the brine. You can also replace the white wine vinegar with white vinegar, red wine vinegar, or apple cider vinegar.

PER SERVING Calories: 32; Total Fat: 0g; Saturated Fat: 0g; Cholesterol: 0mg; Carbohydrates: 5g; Fiber: 1g; Protein: 1g

ZUCCHINI "HUMMUS" WITH CARROT STICKS

Serves 4 / Prep time: 15 minutes

Traditional chickpea hummus is out, but this delicious recipe allows you to experience the tasty Mediterranean flavors of hummus while still maintaining your healthy way of eating. Dip baby carrot sticks in the hummus. If you don't have problems with nightshades, you can also use sliced red bell peppers as a dipping medium.

NIGHTSHADE-FREE

NUT-FREE

VEGAN

MAKE-AHEAD

QUICK & EASY

2 garlic cloves
¼ cup tahini (sesame seed paste)
Juice of 1 lemon
½ teaspoon ground cumin
½ teaspoon sea salt
1 medium zucchini, peeled and cut into pieces
2 tablespoons extra-virgin olive oil, divided
1 pound baby carrots

1. Chop the garlic cloves, then add to the bowl of a food processor, along with the tahini, lemon juice, cumin, and salt. Blend until combined, about 30 seconds.

2. Scrape down the sides of the food processor. Add the zucchini and 1 tablespoon of olive oil. Process until the zucchini is smooth, about 1 minute.

3. Scrape the hummus into a bowl, and drizzle with the remaining 1 tablespoon olive oil.

4. Serve with baby carrots for dipping.

PER SERVING Calories: 200; Total Fat: 15g; Saturated Fat: 2g; Cholesterol: 0mg; Carbohydrates: 15g; Fiber: 5g; Protein: 4g

ZUCCHINI ROUNDS with TAPENADE

Serves 4 / Prep time: 15 minutes

Tapenade is a simple spread made with black olives and seasoning. While traditionally tapenade is spread on crusty bread, here you spread it on thin zucchini slices. It's a delicious way to use the abundance of zucchini as it comes into season in the late summer and early autumn.

1 cup black olives, rinsed, pitted, and chopped
Juice of 1 lemon
¼ cup fresh Italian parsley
1 garlic clove
2 tablespoons extra-virgin olive oil
1 medium zucchini, sliced into ¼-inch rounds

1. In the bowl of a food processor, combine the olives, lemon juice, parsley, garlic, and olive oil.

2. Pulse the food processor for 10 one-second pulses, until all the ingredients are chopped and blended.

3. Serve the tapenade spooned on top of the zucchini rounds.

PER SERVING Calories: 109; Total Fat: 11g; Saturated Fat: 2g; Cholesterol: 0mg; Carbohydrates: 4g; Fiber: 2g; Protein: 1g

NIGHTSHADE-FREE

NUT-FREE

VEGAN

MAKE-AHEAD

QUICK & EASY

GUACAMOLE WITH JICAMA

Serves 4 / Prep time: 15 minutes

If you make this guacamole ahead of time, you can keep it from turning brown by storing it properly. Put it in a bowl, and cover it with plastic wrap. Press the plastic wrap directly down on the surface of the guacamole so no air can get to it. Refrigerate for up to twenty-four hours before serving.

NUT-FREE

VEGAN

MAKE-AHEAD

QUICK &
EASY

2 avocados, peeled, pitted, and cut into cubes

Juice of 1 lime

2 garlic cloves, minced

½ red onion, minced

¼ cup fresh cilantro, finely chopped

½ teaspoon sea salt

1 jicama, peeled and cut into slices

1. In a medium bowl, using a fork, mash the avocados. Mix together with the lime juice, garlic, onion, cilantro, and salt.

2. Serve the guacamole with the jicama slices for dipping.

PER SERVING Calories: 277; Total Fat: 20g; Saturated Fat: 4g; Cholesterol: 0mg; Carbohydrates: 25g; Fiber: 15g; Protein: 3g

AVOCADO DEVILED EGGS

Serves 8 / Prep time: 10 minutes / Cook time: 10 minutes

Deviled eggs are super easy to make, and they are quite filling. Plus, you can make them well ahead of time and take them with you as an appetizer or snack. They even make a delicious lunch or breakfast, if you don't have time to prepare anything else. Make sure when you choose Dijon mustard, you find one without wheat flour. Grey Poupon Dijon is a good brand that doesn't have any gluten in it.

8 eggs, hardboiled (page 233)
¼ cup Homemade Mayonnaise (page 229)
½ avocado, peeled, pitted, and mashed
Juice of ½ lemon
1 tablespoon Dijon mustard
½ teaspoon sea salt
¼ teaspoon freshly ground black pepper

1. Peel the cooled eggs, and slice them lengthwise. Remove the yolks with a teaspoon, and put them in a small bowl. Put the whites, cut-side up, on a platter.

2. Add the Homemade Mayonnaise, avocado, lemon juice, mustard, salt, and pepper to the bowl with the yolks.

3. Mash the ingredients together with a fork until they are well blended.

4. Spoon the yolk mixture back into the egg halves and serve.

Ingredient tip: Hardboiled eggs are easier to peel when they are about a week old. Fresh eggs are notoriously difficult to peel, so use older eggs. To ease peeling, run the eggs under cold water as you peel them.

PER SERVING Calories: 119; Total Fat: 9g; Saturated Fat: 2g; Cholesterol: 166mg; Carbohydrates: 3g; Fiber: 1g; Protein: 6g

NIGHTSHADE-FREE

NUT-FREE

VEGETARIAN

MAKE-AHEAD

QUICK & EASY

BABA GANOUSH WITH ROMAINE LETTUCE BOATS

Serves 4 / Prep time: 10 minutes / Cook time: 10 minutes

The main ingredient in this dish is eggplant. If you have a sensitivity to nightshades, avoid this snack and have another instead. This baba ganoush is seasoned with typical Mediterranean flavors of lemon and garlic. Use the inner leaves of the romaine to make boats to hold the dip. If you make this recipe ahead of time, wait to scoop it into the lettuce leaves until just before serving.

1 eggplant, peeled and cut into ¼-inch-thick rounds
Sea salt
Juice of 1 lemon
2 garlic cloves, minced
1 tablespoon tahini
3 tablespoons extra-virgin olive oil, divided
½ teaspoon sea salt
¼ teaspoon freshly ground black pepper
8 romaine lettuce leaves
2 tablespoons chopped fresh Italian parsley

1. Sprinkle the eggplant rounds with salt, and place them in a colander in the sink. Let them sit for 10 minutes so the bitter juices can drain away.

2. Preheat the broiler to high.

3. Rinse and dry the eggplant rounds.

4. Place the eggplant rounds on a broiler pan and put them under the broiler.

5. Broil, turning the eggplant once or twice in the process, until the rounds are soft and golden brown, about 7 minutes.

6. Remove the eggplant from the oven, and put it in the bowl of a food processor along with the lemon juice, garlic, tahini, 2 tablespoons of olive oil, and the salt and pepper. Blend until everything is smooth and combined, about 30 seconds.

7. Scoop the baba ganoush into the lettuce leaves and drizzle with the remaining 1 tablespoon olive oil.

8. Sprinkle with the parsley and serve.

Ingredient tip: Salting the eggplant and allowing it to drain for about 10 minutes helps remove the bitter juices, making your dip tastier.

PER SERVING Calories: 145; Total Fat: 13g; Saturated Fat: 2g; Cholesterol: 0mg; Carbohydrates: 8g; Fiber: 5g; Protein: 2g

SALMON SALAD WITH CUCUMBER ROUNDS

Serves 4 / Prep time: 10 minutes

Use canned or cooked fresh salmon for this recipe. Be sure to use wild-caught salmon and not farmed salmon, which may be high in potentially harmful chemicals called PCBs. You can also use smoked salmon or smoked trout in this recipe.

NIGHTSHADE-FREE

NUT-FREE

MAKE-AHEAD

QUICK & EASY

8 ounces wild-caught salmon, cooked

½ cup Homemade Mayonnaise (page 229)

1 tablespoon Dijon mustard

1 tablespoon chopped fresh dill

Zest of 1 lemon

1 celery stalk, finely chopped

½ teaspoon sea salt

¼ teaspoon freshly ground black pepper

1 medium cucumber, cut into ¼-inch rounds

1. In a medium bowl, stir together the salmon, Homemade Mayonnaise, mustard, dill, lemon zest, celery, salt, and pepper until well mixed.

2. Spoon the salmon salad onto the cucumber rounds and serve.

Substitution tip: Try this recipe with cooked baby shrimp instead of salmon.

PER SERVING Calories: 217; Total Fat: 14g; Saturated Fat: 2g; Cholesterol: 33mg; Carbohydrates: 11g; Fiber: 1g; Protein: 13g

SHRIMP SALAD with AVOCADO

Serves 2 / Prep time: 10 minutes

WEEK 2

This is an easy snack to make ahead and take with you. Keep it chilled in a tightly sealed container. The fats in the salad and the avocado are very satisfying, so it can also serve as a light lunch or dinner.

○ NIGHTSHADE-FREE

○ NUT-FREE

○ MAKE-AHEAD

○ QUICK & EASY

6 ounces wild-caught bay shrimp, cooked

⅓ cup Homemade Mayonnaise (page 229)

Juice and zest of 1 lemon

2 scallions, finely chopped

1 celery stalk, finely chopped

½ teaspoon sea salt

¼ teaspoon freshly ground black pepper

1 avocado, halved and pitted

1. In a medium bowl, stir together the shrimp, Homemade Mayonnaise, lemon juice, lemon zest, scallions, celery, salt, and pepper until well mixed.

2. Using a large spoon, scoop the avocado halves out of their peel. Rub the avocado with the squeezed lemon halves.

3. Place the avocado halves cut-side up on two plates, scoop the shrimp salad into the avocado halves, and serve.

PER SERVING Calories: 492; Total Fat: 41g; Saturated Fat: 8g; Cholesterol: 189mg; Carbohydrates: 11g; Fiber: 7g; Protein: 22g

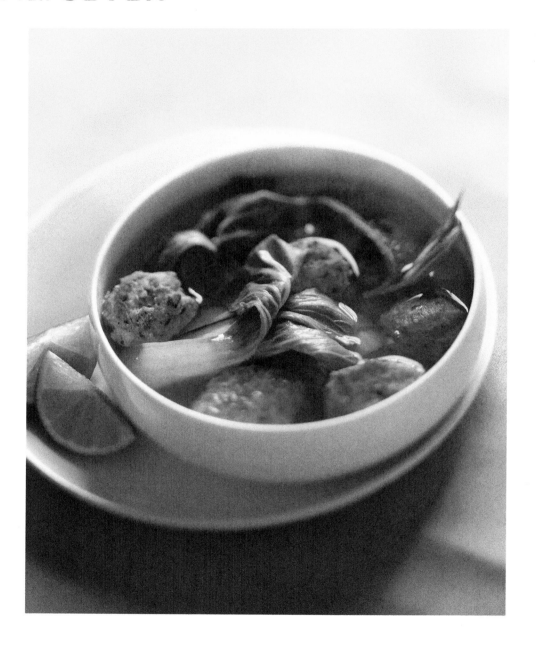

SOUPS AND STEWS

SUMMER GAZPACHO

Serves 4 / Prep time: 10 minutes

This chilled soup is refreshing for a light summer lunch or dinner. It is at its most delicious during the summer, when tomatoes and fresh herbs are in season. While you can use any farm-fresh tomatoes, tender cherry tomatoes or delicious heirloom tomatoes offer a sweetness that can't be beat. For a sweet onion, try a Vidalia or Walla Walla variety.

NUT-FREE

VEGAN

QUICK &
EASY

4 large heirloom tomatoes, chopped

1 large cucumber, seeded and peeled

1 sweet onion, chopped

2 garlic cloves, chopped

1 cup tomato juice

Juice of 1 lemon

2 tablespoons extra-virgin olive oil

Dash cayenne pepper

½ teaspoon sea salt

¼ teaspoon freshly ground black pepper

4 large basil leaves, cut into a chiffonade

1. In a blender or food processor, blend the tomatoes, cucumber, onion, garlic, tomato juice, lemon juice, olive oil, cayenne, salt, and pepper until the mixture is smooth.

2. Serve chilled, garnished with the basil.

Cooking Tip: Chiffonade means cut into long, thin strips. To cut basil into a chiffonade, stack the basil leaves and roll them into a loose roll. Then, using a sharp knife, cut the roll into thin strips.

PER SERVING Calories: 234; Total Fat: 25g; Saturated Fat: 2g; Cholesterol: 0mg; Carbohydrates: 26g; Fiber: 5g; Protein: 5g

MUSHROOM, FENNEL, AND ITALIAN SAUSAGE SOUP

Serves 6 / Prep time: 20 minutes / Cook time: 25 minutes

WEEK 1 / WEEK 4

If you can find sugar-free bulk Italian sausage at the grocery store, you can save yourself a step and use it in this recipe. Otherwise, you'll need to make your own Italian sausage. The process is pretty easy, and the flavorful results are worthwhile.

NIGHTSHADE-
FREE

NUT-FREE

MAKE-AHEAD

1 pound Italian Sausage (page 234)

1 onion, chopped

1 fennel bulb, thinly sliced

4 garlic cloves, minced

8 cups Slow Cooker Bone Broth (page 226)

8 ounces cremini mushrooms, sliced

3 carrots, sliced

1. In a large soup pot over medium-high heat, cook the Italian Sausage, crumbling with a spoon, until it is cooked through, about 5 minutes. Remove the sausage from the rendered fat with a slotted spoon and set it aside.

2. Add the onion and fennel to the fat in the pot. Cook, stirring occasionally, for about 4 minutes. Add the garlic and continue to cook, stirring, until the vegetables are soft, about 1 more minute.

3. Add the Slow Cooker Bone Broth, mushrooms, carrots, and reserved sausage to the pan. Cook until the carrots and mushrooms are soft, about 10 minutes.

PER SERVING Calories: 340; Total Fat: 23g; Saturated Fat: 7g; Cholesterol: 64mg; Carbohydrates: 8g; Fiber: 2g; Protein: 23g

CHICKEN SOUP WITH ZUCCHINI "NOODLES"

Serves 6 / Prep time: 10 minutes / Cook time: 20 minutes

NIGHTSHADE-
FREE

NUT-FREE

MAKE-AHEAD

QUICK &
EASY

You can make this soup ahead of time and freeze it for quick lunches or dinners on nights when you just don't have the time to cook. Cut the zucchini in long, thin noodle shapes with a knife, a mandoline, or a spiralizer.

2 tablespoons coconut oil

1 pound boneless, skinless chicken thighs, cut into ½-inch pieces

1 onion, chopped

2 celery stalks, chopped

2 carrots, peeled and chopped

3 garlic cloves, minced

8 cups Slow Cooker Bone Broth (page 226)

1 teaspoon dried thyme

½ teaspoon sea salt

½ teaspoon freshly ground black pepper

1 medium zucchini, cut into "noodles"

1. In a large soup pot over medium-high heat, heat the coconut oil until it shimmers. Add the chicken and cook, stirring frequently, until the chicken is cooked through, 6 to 8 minutes. Remove the chicken from the oil with a slotted spoon and set it aside on a platter.

2. In the remaining oil, cook the onion, celery, and carrots, stirring occasionally, until the vegetables are soft, about 5 minutes.

3. Add the garlic and cook, stirring constantly, until it is fragrant, about 30 seconds.

4. Add the Slow Cooker Bone Broth, scraping any browned bits from the bottom of the pot with a spoon.

5. Add the thyme, salt, pepper, reserved chicken, and any juices that have collected on the platter. Bring the mixture to a boil, and reduce the heat to simmer.

6. Add the zucchini "noodles," cook until the zucchini is soft, 3 to 4 more minutes, and serve.

PER SERVING Calories: 258; Total Fat: 12g; Saturated Fat: 6g; Cholesterol: 67mg; Carbohydrates: 7g; Fiber: 1g; Protein: 29g

COCONUT SHRIMP CHOWDER

Serves 6 / Prep time: 10 minutes / Cook time: 25 minutes

WEEK 1 / WEEK 3

This hearty chowder makes a wonderful dinner. It also freezes well, so you can make it ahead and take it for lunches or a quick dinner during the week. The shrimp here should be 36 to 40 count. Count refers to the number of individual shrimp in a pound, so the bigger the number, the smaller the shrimp.

NIGHTSHADE-FREE

NUT-FREE

MAKE-AHEAD

2 tablespoons coconut oil

1 onion, chopped

4 garlic cloves, minced

Juice of 2 limes

6 cups Slow Cooker Bone Broth (page 226)

1 sweet potato, peeled and cut into ½-inch cubes

3 large carrots, peeled and sliced

1 (14-ounce) can coconut milk

½ teaspoon sea salt

½ teaspoon freshly ground black pepper

1 pound shrimp, peeled, deveined, and tails removed

¼ cup arrowroot powder

¼ cup water

1. In a large soup pot over medium-high heat, heat the coconut oil until it shimmers. Add the onion and cook, stirring occasionally, until it starts to brown, about 5 minutes.

2. Add the garlic cloves and cook, stirring constantly, until the garlic is fragrant, about 30 seconds.

3. Add the lime juice and Slow Cooker Bone Broth, scraping any browned bits from the bottom of the pan with a spoon.

4. Add the sweet potato, carrots, coconut milk, salt, and pepper, and bring to a simmer. Reduce the heat to medium and simmer until the potatoes are soft, about 10 minutes.

5. Add the shrimp and cook until they turn pink, 3 to 4 minutes more.

6. In a small bowl, whisk together the arrowroot powder and water. Add it to the soup pot and bring to a simmer, stirring constantly.

7. Cook until the soup thickens slightly, about 4 minutes, and serve.

PER SERVING Calories: 423; Total Fat: 26g; Saturated Fat: 22g; Cholesterol: 153mg; Carbohydrates: 23g; Fiber: 4g; Protein: 25g

ASIAN MEATBALL SOUP

Serves 6 / Prep time: 10 minutes / Cook time: 25 minutes

This flavorful soup is filled with delicious vegetables. Then you cook the pork meatballs in the soup for even more flavor. This soup freezes well, so it's a great make-ahead recipe. You can even make and freeze the meatballs and soup separately, and then cook them together when you're hungry.

MAKE-AHEAD

FOR THE SOUP

2 tablespoons coconut oil

1 onion, chopped

4 garlic cloves, minced

1 tablespoon fresh grated ginger

8 cups Slow Cooker Bone Broth (page 226)

1 tablespoon coconut aminos

½ teaspoon sea salt

½ teaspoon freshly ground black pepper

1 cup baby bok choy

1 lime, sliced into wedges

FOR THE MEATBALLS

1 pound ground pork

2 garlic cloves, minced

2 tablespoons chopped fresh cilantro

1 egg, beaten

1 tablespoon coconut aminos

½ cup almond flour

1 tablespoon fresh grated ginger

½ teaspoon sea salt

½ teaspoon freshly ground black pepper

TO MAKE THE SOUP

1. In a large soup pot over medium-high heat, heat the coconut oil until it shimmers. Add the onion and cook, stirring occasionally, until it is soft, about 5 minutes.

2. Add the garlic and ginger, and cook, stirring constantly, until the garlic is fragrant, about 30 seconds.

3. Add the Slow Cooker Bone Broth, coconut aminos, salt, pepper, and bok choy. Bring the soup to a simmer, and reduce the heat to medium.

TO MAKE THE MEATBALLS

1. In a large bowl, mix the ground pork, garlic, cilantro, egg, coconut aminos, flour, ginger, salt, and pepper until well combined.

2. Shape the mixture into ½-inch meatballs, and drop them into the simmering soup. Cover and cook until the meatballs are cooked through, about 15 minutes.

3. Ladle into bowls and serve with a wedge of lime.

Ingredient tip: This recipe calls for coconut aminos, which is made from coconut sap and is often used as a soy sauce substitute. It can be found in many large grocery store chains and health food stores, or online. You can also use Bragg's liquid aminos in place of the coconut aminos, if you wish. Bragg's is made from soybeans, though, so if this is one of the foods you can't tolerate, stick with the coconut version.

PER SERVING Calories: 322; Total Fat: 15g; Saturated Fat: 6g; Cholesterol: 82mg; Carbohydrates: 14g; Fiber: 4g; Protein: 29g

GROUND BEEF AND VEGETABLE SOUP

Serves 4 / Prep time: 10 minutes / Cook time: 20 minutes

WEEK 2 / WEEK 4

Ground beef makes a versatile base for a soup. You can mix it up by adding any vegetables you wish. If you find you tolerate nightshades well, you can zip up this soup with a can of crushed tomatoes and a pinch of red pepper flakes.

NIGHTSHADE-
FREE

NUT-FREE

MAKE-AHEAD

QUICK &
EASY

2 tablespoons coconut oil

1 pound ground beef

1 onion, chopped

3 garlic cloves, minced

6 cups Slow Cooker Bone Broth (page 226)

2 carrots, chopped

1 zucchini, chopped

8 ounces green beans, chopped

8 ounces button mushrooms, sliced

½ teaspoon sea salt

½ teaspoon freshly ground black pepper

1 teaspoon dried thyme

1. In a large soup pot over medium-high heat, heat the coconut oil until it shimmers. Add the ground beef and cook, crumbling it with a spoon, until it is browned, about 5 minutes.

2. Add the onions and cook, stirring occasionally, until the onions are soft, about 5 minutes.

3. Add the garlic and cook, stirring constantly, until the garlic is fragrant, about 30 seconds.

4. Add the Slow Cooker Bone Broth, scraping any browned bits from the bottom of the pan with a spoon.

5. Add the carrots, zucchini, green beans, mushrooms, salt, pepper, and thyme.

6. Bring the soup to a simmer, stirring occasionally, and reduce the heat to medium.

7. Continue simmering until the vegetables are soft, about 10 minutes more, and serve.

Time-saving tip: Save chopping time by using a bag of frozen organic mixed vegetables instead of the fresh vegetables. Just be sure the vegetable mix you use doesn't have added chemicals, nightshades, or corn.

PER SERVING Calories: 434; Total Fat: 16g; Saturated Fat: 9g; Cholesterol: 101mg; Carbohydrates: 24g; Fiber: 8g; Protein: 48g

SLOW COOKER BEANLESS CHILI

Serves 8 / Prep time: 20 minutes / Cook time: 8 hours

Using a combination of ground beef and ground pork adds interesting flavors and textures to this beanless chili. You can adjust the spiciness of the chili by adding more or less cayenne pepper. If you are sensitive to nightshades, don't eat this dish.

NUT-FREE

MAKE-AHEAD

1 pound ground beef

1 pound ground pork

1 onion, chopped

1 jalapeño pepper, seeded and minced

1 green bell pepper, seeded and chopped

2 (15-ounce) cans crushed tomatoes, undrained

2 cups Slow Cooker Bone Broth (page 226)

1 tablespoon chili powder

1 teaspoon ground cumin

1 teaspoon dried oregano

½ teaspoon ground coriander

1 teaspoon sea salt

½ teaspoon freshly ground black pepper

⅛ teaspoon ground cayenne pepper

1 avocado, peeled, pitted, and chopped

1. In a large sauté pan, working in batches, brown the ground beef and ground pork, crumbling it with a spoon as it cooks. Drain the fat, and add the meat to the slow cooker.

2. Add the onion, jalapeño, green pepper, tomatoes, Slow Cooker Bone Broth, chili powder, cumin, oregano, coriander, salt, pepper, and cayenne to the slow cooker and stir it well.

3. Cover the slow cooker, and turn it on low. Cook for 8 hours.

4. Garnish with the avocado slices and serve.

PER SERVING Calories: 298; Total Fat: 11g; Saturated Fat: 3g; Cholesterol: 92mg; Carbohydrates: 13g; Fiber: 6g; Protein: 37g

SLOW COOKER PORK CHILI COLORADO

Serves 8 / Prep time: 20 minutes / Cook time: 8 hours

Use pork shoulder in this recipe, an inexpensive cut that retains its flavor and texture in the slow cooker. This is the perfect dish for a winter's evening. It only takes about twenty minutes in the morning to get this dish ready, and you'll come home after work to a delicious-smelling house and a hearty meal. This freezes well too. Serve topped with homemade Guacamole (page 106).

NUT-FREE

MAKE-AHEAD

1 dried chipotle chile

1 dried New Mexico chile

½ teaspoon ground cumin

½ teaspoon dried oregano

1 teaspoon garlic powder

1 teaspoon onion powder

1 teaspoon sea salt

1 teaspoon freshly ground black pepper

3 pounds pastured pork shoulder, cut into 1-inch chunks

1 onion, chopped

3 garlic cloves, chopped

2 cups Slow Cooker Bone Broth (page 226)

1. In the bowl of a food processor fitted with a chopping blade, pulse the chipotle and New Mexico chiles for 20 one-second pulses, until they form a powder.

2. Add the cumin, oregano, garlic powder, onion powder, salt, and pepper to the food processor. Pulse for 10 one-second pulses to combine.

3. In a slow cooker, stir together the pork shoulder, onion, garlic, Slow Cooker Bone Broth, and the chile and spice mixture.

4. Cover the slow cooker, and turn it on low.

5. Cook for 8 hours, or until the pork is tender, and serve.

PER SERVING Calories: 376; Total Fat: 27g; Saturated Fat: 9g; Cholesterol: 120mg; Carbohydrates: 2g; Fiber: 0g; Protein: 31g

SLOW COOKER BEEF STEW

Serves 8 / Prep time: 20 minutes / Cook time: 8 hours

NIGHTSHADE-
FREE

NUT-FREE

MAKE-AHEAD

Chuck roast is one of the best types of meat for the long, slow braise you get with a slow cooker. This hearty stew is a great winter dish, because it makes the most of seasonal vegetables you'll find in the fall and winter. Celeriac makes a great substitute for potatoes.

2 pounds beef chuck roast, cut into 1-inch pieces

1 large onion, chopped

3 garlic cloves, chopped

3 cups Slow Cooker Bone Broth (page 226)

¼ cup balsamic vinegar

1 teaspoon dried thyme

1 teaspoon dried rosemary

2 bulbs celeriac, peeled and cut into ½-inch cubes

4 carrots, peeled and cut into chunks

2 celery stalks, chopped

8 ounces cremini mushrooms, quartered

1 teaspoon sea salt

½ teaspoon freshly ground black pepper

½ cup arrowroot powder

½ cup water

1. In a slow cooker, stir together the beef, onion, garlic, Slow Cooker Bone Broth, vinegar, thyme, rosemary, celeriac, carrots, celery, mushrooms, salt, and pepper.

2. In a small bowl, whisk together the arrowroot powder and the water until well combined. Add to the slow cooker and stir all the ingredients to mix them.

3. Cook, covered, on low heat for 8 to 10 hours, until the beef is tender, and serve.

Substitution tip: Celeriac, which is also called celery root, has a hearty vegetable flavor that is like a cross between celery and parsley. Peel the knobby, bulbous root with a sharp knife and use it right away, because, just like with a potato, the cut surfaces will darken.

PER SERVING Calories: 325; Total Fat: 10g; Saturated Fat: 4g; Cholesterol: 115mg; Carbohydrates: 17g; Fiber: 2g; Protein: 39g

SLOW COOKER JAMBALAYA

Serves 8 / Prep time: 20 minutes / Cook time: 8 hours

While this New Orleans favorite is typically made with rice, here it is more of a stew. Many brands of andouille sausage are sugar-free and gluten-free. Check the manufacturer's website to make sure you purchase a gluten-free brand. This is a great dinner option post-plan if you find that your body has no reaction to tomatoes and grains such as rice.

NUT-FREE

MAKE-AHEAD

3 slices bacon, cut into pieces

1 pound boneless, skinless chicken thighs, cut into 1-inch pieces

1 pound andouille sausage, cut into 1-inch pieces

1 onion, chopped

1 red bell pepper, seeded and chopped

1 green bell pepper, seeded and chopped

1 yellow bell pepper, seeded and chopped

2 cups Slow Cooker Bone Broth (page 226)

1 (15-ounce) can crushed tomatoes, undrained

1 teaspoon dried oregano

1 teaspoon dried thyme

1 teaspoon dried basil

⅛ teaspoon ground cayenne pepper

1 teaspoon sea salt

½ teaspoon freshly ground black pepper

1 pound shrimp, peeled, deveined, tails removed

Juice of 1 lemon

1. In a large sauté pan over medium-high heat, cook the bacon until it is browned. Put the bacon and the rendered fat in the slow cooker.

2. Add the chicken, andouille, onion, red pepper, green pepper, yellow pepper, Slow Cooker Bone Broth, tomatoes, oregano, thyme, basil, cayenne, salt, and pepper to the slow cooker.

3. Cover the slow cooker, and turn it on low. Cook for 7 hours.

4. Add the shrimp and lemon juice to the slow cooker, and increase the heat to high.

5. Cook, covered, for 1 more hour, until the shrimp are pink, and serve.

PER SERVING Calories: 460; Total Fat: 24g; Saturated Fat: 8g; Cholesterol: 210mg; Carbohydrates: 13g; Fiber: 3g; Protein: 46g

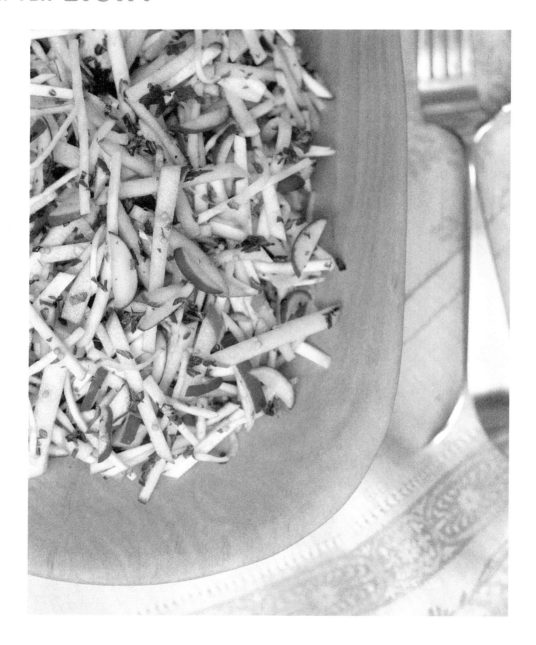

CHAPTER EIGHT

SALADS

POMEGRANATE, BLACKBERRY, AND SATSUMA SALAD

Serves 4 / Prep time: 10 minutes

NIGHTSHADE-FREE

NUT-FREE

MAKE-AHEAD

QUICK & EASY

In the late fall you can find the last of the blackberries and the first of the pomegranates and satsuma oranges. The tiny oranges are flavorful and easy to peel, and the sections are the perfect bite size for a salad. This is a great salad to go with fall meals.

8 satsuma oranges, peeled and sectioned

1 cup pomegranate seeds, thin white covering removed

2 cups blackberries

1. In a medium bowl, toss together the satsuma sections, pomegranate arils, and blackberries.

2. Serve immediately, or chill, covered, for up to 8 hours.

PER SERVING Calories: 189; Total Fat: .3g; Saturated Fat: 0g; Cholesterol: 0mg; Carbohydrates: 43g; Fiber: 7g; Protein: 3g

APPLE AND GINGER SLAW

Serves 4 / Prep time: 10 minutes

WEEK 1 / WEEK 4

Add a little sweetness to a traditional coleslaw recipe by adding Granny Smith apples, which are sweet-tart. You can also try other sweet-tart apples, such as Honeycrisp or Pink Lady. While cabbage is a goitrogen, a small amount is fine on a Hashimoto's diet. Serve this recipe in the fall when apples and cabbage are at their peak.

2 sweet-tart apples, peeled, cored, and julienned
8 radishes, julienned
3 tablespoons freshly chopped cilantro
1 tablespoon fresh grated ginger
1 tablespoon apple cider vinegar
½ cup Homemade Mayonnaise (page 229)
½ teaspoon sea salt
¼ teaspoon freshly ground black pepper

1. In a large bowl, combine the apples, radishes, and cilantro.

2. In a small bowl, whisk together the ginger, vinegar, Homemade Mayonnaise, salt, and pepper.

3. Toss the dressing with the salad. Serve immediately or refrigerate for up to 12 hours.

Substitution tip: Try replacing half the apples with a julienned cucumber for a uniquely refreshing slaw.

PER SERVING Calories: 212; Total Fat: 10g; Saturated Fat: 1g; Cholesterol: 8mg; Carbohydrates: 33g; Fiber: 6g; Protein: 1g

○
NIGHTSHADE-FREE

○
NUT-FREE

○
MAKE-AHEAD

○
QUICK & EASY

ARUGULA, PEAR, FIG, AND WALNUT SALAD

Serves 6 / Prep time: 10 minutes

Fresh figs have two harvest seasons: early summer and early fall. That's because fig trees produce two distinct crops of fruit every year. The fresh figs—distinctly different from dried figs—add a delicate sweetness and a little crunch to this wonderful seasonal salad.

FOR THE VINAIGRETTE

2 tablespoons balsamic vinegar

2 tablespoons walnut oil

2 tablespoons extra-virgin olive oil

¼ teaspoon Dijon mustard

¼ teaspoon sea salt

¼ teaspoon freshly ground black pepper

FOR THE SALAD

1 pint fresh figs, stemmed and quartered

1 pear, peeled, cored, and sliced

6 cups arugula

½ cup chopped walnuts

TO MAKE THE VINAIGRETTE

In a small bowl, whisk together the vinegar, walnut oil, olive oil, mustard, salt, and pepper.

TO MAKE THE SALAD

1. In a large bowl, combine the figs, pears, arugula, and walnuts.

2. Toss the salad with the dressing, and serve immediately.

Cooking tip: If you make this salad ahead, don't toss it with the dressing until just before you serve it.

PER SERVING Calories: 305; Total Fat: 13g; Saturated Fat: 1g; Cholesterol: 0mg; Carbohydrates: 48g; Fiber: 9g; Protein: 6g

JICAMA, ZUCCHINI, AND AVOCADO SLAW

Serves 4 / Prep time: 10 minutes

WEEK 2

Serve this slaw with a grilled chicken breast or a delicious fish fillet. You can find jicama in the grocery store produce section. Peel it and cut it into a very thin julienne. This recipe is a great way to use the copious amounts of zucchini that turn up in gardens from late summer to early fall.

1 jicama, peeled and julienned or grated

2 medium zucchini, peeled and julienned or grated

1 avocado, peeled and pitted

2 tablespoons apple cider vinegar

Juice and zest of 1 lemon

1 garlic clove, minced

½ teaspoon sea salt

½ teaspoon freshly ground black pepper

1. In a large bowl, stir together the jicama and zucchini.

2. In the bowl of a blender or food processor, process the avocado, vinegar, lemon juice, lemon zest, garlic, salt, and pepper for 30 seconds to 1 minute to combine.

3. Toss the avocado dressing with the slaw, and serve immediately.

PER SERVING Calories: 122; Total Fat: 10g; Saturated Fat: 2g; Cholesterol: 0mg; Carbohydrates: 8g; Fiber: 5g; Protein: 2g

NIGHTSHADE-FREE

NUT-FREE

MAKE-AHEAD

QUICK & EASY

SPINACH SALAD WITH WARM BACON VINAIGRETTE

Serves 4 / Prep time: 10 minutes / Cook time: 10 minutes

WEEK 2

NIGHTSHADE-FREE

NUT-FREE

QUICK & EASY

The warm bacon vinaigrette adds a smoky flavor to the spinach that is irresistible. Enjoy this salad by itself or as an accompaniment to a nice cut of meat. Use fresh baby spinach for the salad, as it has the best texture and flavor when combined with the vinaigrette.

6 cups baby spinach
4 slices bacon, cut into pieces
½ cup red wine vinegar
1 tablespoon minced shallots
3 garlic cloves, minced
¼ teaspoon sea salt
¼ teaspoon freshly ground black pepper

1. Put the spinach in a large bowl.

2. In a large sauté pan over medium-high heat, cook the bacon until it is crisp and the fat is rendered. Using a slotted spoon, remove the bacon from the rendered fat and blot it with paper towels. Put it in the bowl with the spinach.

3. Remove and set aside all but 2 tablespoons of bacon fat from the sauté pan. In the sauté pan, still over medium-high heat, simmer the vinegar, shallots, garlic, salt, and pepper until the liquid reduces to about ¼ cup.

4. Pour the warm dressing over the spinach and bacon, toss to combine, and serve immediately.

PER SERVING Calories: 226; Total Fat: 20g; Saturated Fat: 8g; Cholesterol: 29mg; Carbohydrates: 3g; Fiber: 1g; Protein: 7g

GREEK SALAD with SHRIMP

Serves 4 / Prep time: 10 minutes

WEEK 1 / WEEK 4

This salad uses cooked bay shrimp, which you should be able to find fresh at the fish counter of your grocery store. If you can't find Kalamata olives, or don't like them, feel free to substitute any olives of your choosing.

2 medium cucumbers, peeled and chopped

1 red onion, thinly sliced

9 ounces baby arugula

¼ cup Kalamata olives, pitted and chopped

½ cup fresh Italian parsley, chopped

1 pound bay shrimp, cooked

¼ cup extra-virgin olive oil

2 tablespoons red wine vinegar

¼ teaspoon dried oregano

½ teaspoon sea salt

¼ teaspoon freshly ground black pepper

1. In a large bowl, toss together the cucumbers, onion, arugula, olives, parsley, and shrimp.

2. In a small bowl, whisk together the olive oil, vinegar, oregano, salt, and pepper.

3. Toss the salad with the dressing, and serve immediately.

Substitution tip: If you like, replace the shrimp with meat from a grocery store rotisserie chicken or precooked turkey breast.

PER SERVING Calories: 280; Total Fat: 15g; Saturated Fat: 2g; Cholesterol: 223mg; Carbohydrates: 13g; Fiber: 3g; Protein: 27g

NIGHTSHADE-FREE

NUT-FREE

QUICK & EASY

SPINACH AND SHRIMP SALAD WITH RASPBERRY VINAIGRETTE

Serves 4 / Prep time: 10 minutes

NIGHTSHADE-FREE

NUT-FREE

QUICK & EASY

Use cooked bay shrimp for this salad to make it quick and easy. This salad is also satisfying enough to serve as a lunch or a light dinner.

FOR THE VINAIGRETTE

½ cup fresh raspberries

Juice of ½ lemon

¼ cup extra-virgin olive oil

2 tablespoons red wine vinegar

Pinch of sea salt

Pinch of freshly ground black pepper

FOR THE SALAD

6 cups baby spinach

1 pound cooked bay shrimp

2 tablespoons chopped fresh basil

TO MAKE THE VINAIGRETTE

1. In a blender or food processor, process the raspberries for 30 seconds. Pour the raspberries into a small bowl.

2. Whisk in the lemon juice, olive oil, vinegar, salt, and pepper, and set aside.

TO MAKE THE SALAD

1. In a large bowl, combine the spinach, shrimp, and basil.

2. Whisk the dressing once more, and toss with the salad just before serving.

PER SERVING Calories: 236; Total Fat: 14g; Saturated Fat: 2g; Cholesterol: 223mg; Carbohydrates: 4g; Fiber: 2g; Protein: 26g

CHICKEN CAESAR SALAD

Serves 4 / Prep time: 10 minutes

This salad comes together quickly because it uses the meat from a precooked rotisserie chicken breast. Double-check with your grocer to ensure they don't inject a solution into their chicken that contains any gluten or sugar.

8 cups romaine lettuce, shredded

8 ounces rotisserie chicken breast, skin removed

2 garlic cloves, minced

Juice of 1 lemon

1 teaspoon Dijon mustard

2 egg yolks

¼ teaspoon sea salt

¼ teaspoon freshly ground black pepper

¾ cup extra-virgin olive oil

NIGHTSHADE-
FREE

NUT-FREE

QUICK &
EASY

1. In a large bowl, toss together the lettuce and rotisserie chicken.

2. In the bowl of a food processor fitted with a chopping blade, begin processing the garlic, lemon juice, mustard, egg yolks, salt, and pepper.

3. Add a drop of oil at a time through the chute of the running food processor for about 10 drops. Then continue to add the oil in a thin stream until it is completely incorporated.

4. Toss the salad with the dressing, and serve immediately.

PER SERVING Calories: 458; Total Fat: 42g; Saturated Fat: 6g; Cholesterol: 153mg; Carbohydrates: 3g; Fiber: 1g; Protein: 20g

ITALIAN CHOPPED CHICKEN SALAD

Serves 4 / Prep time: 10 minutes

Use precooked rotisserie chicken with the skin removed for this recipe. The chicken thighs work particularly well because they hold up to the bold flavors of the vegetables. For this salad, be sure to buy artichoke hearts packed in water only.

NUT-FREE

MAKE-AHEAD

QUICK & EASY

2 cooked chicken thighs, skin and bones removed, meat chopped

½ red onion, minced

1 red bell pepper, seeded and chopped

2 tomatoes, seeded and chopped

1 cucumber, chopped

1 cup water-packed artichoke hearts, chopped

6 large basil leaves, chopped

½ cup black olives, pitted and chopped

1 green bell pepper, seeded and chopped

½ cup extra-virgin olive oil

¼ cup red wine vinegar

1 tablespoon Dijon mustard

1 garlic clove, minced

¼ teaspoon sea salt

¼ teaspoon freshly ground black pepper

1. In a large bowl, toss together the chicken, onion, red pepper, tomatoes, cucumber, artichoke hearts, basil, olives, and green pepper.

2. In a small bowl, whisk together the olive oil, vinegar, mustard, garlic, salt, and pepper.

3. Pour the dressing over the salad, and toss to combine. Serve immediately, or refrigerate for up to 4 hours.

PER SERVING Calories: 422; Total Fat: 31g; Saturated Fat: 5g; Cholesterol: 62mg; Carbohydrates: 15g; Fiber: 5g; Protein: 24g

EGG SALAD in BUTTER LETTUCE CUPS

Serves 4 / Prep time: 10 minutes

3-DAY CLEANSE / WEEK 2 / WEEK 3

Hard-boiling eggs takes about twenty minutes from start to finish. Alternatively, many grocery stores have now started to sell pre-peeled hardboiled eggs. You can follow the recipe for Hardboiled Eggs (page 233), or you can save time by purchasing them already peeled.

8 hardboiled eggs, peeled and chopped
3 scallions, chopped
1 tablespoon Dijon mustard
¼ cup Homemade Mayonnaise (page 229)
¼ teaspoon sea salt
¼ teaspoon freshly ground black pepper
4 large butter lettuce leaves

○ NIGHTSHADE-FREE

○ NUT-FREE

○ MAKE-AHEAD

○ QUICK & EASY

1. In a large bowl, stir together the eggs and scallions.

2. In a small bowl, whisk together the mustard, Homemade Mayonnaise, salt, and pepper.

3. Gently fold the mayonnaise mixture into the egg mixture.

4. Spoon the egg salad into the lettuce leaves, and serve immediately.

PER SERVING Calories: 192; Total Fat: 14g; Saturated Fat: 4g; Cholesterol: 31mg; Carbohydrates: 6g; Fiber: 1g; Protein: 12g

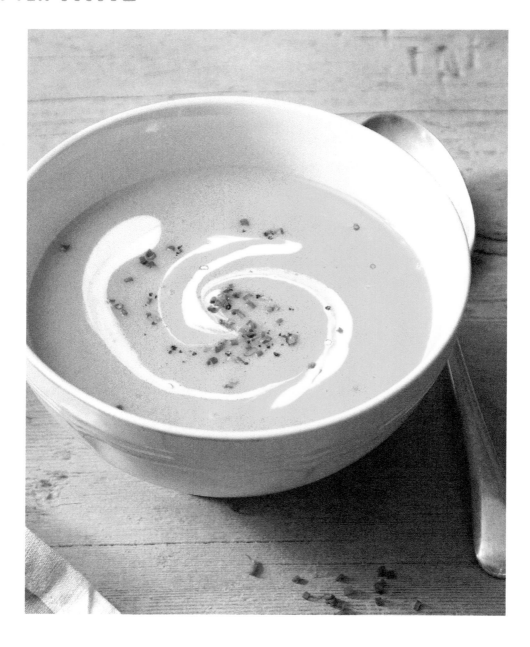

CHAPTER NINE

VEGETARIAN DINNERS

VEGETABLE STIR-FRY WITH CAULIFLOWER "RICE"

Serves 4 / Prep time: 10 minutes / Cook time: 20 minutes

WEEK 3

NIGHTSHADE-
FREE

NUT-FREE

VEGAN

QUICK &
EASY

Finely chopped cauliflower takes the place of rice in this quick and easy stir-fry. If you'd like, you can make the "rice" ahead of time and freeze it raw. Then, cook it from frozen as you prepare the stir-fry. You can use any vegetables you like in this stir-fry.

2 tablespoons coconut oil

½ onion, sliced

2 carrots, peeled and sliced

8 ounces shiitake mushrooms, sliced

1 medium zucchini, sliced

1 cup broccoli florets

3 scallions, sliced

1 tablespoon fresh grated ginger

3 garlic cloves, minced

2 tablespoons coconut aminos

2 tablespoons rice vinegar

2 tablespoons arrowroot powder

1 recipe Cauliflower "Rice" (page 231)

1. In a large sauté pan or wok over medium-high heat, heat the coconut oil until it shimmers.

2. Add the onion, carrots, mushrooms, zucchini, broccoli, scallions, and ginger. Cook, stirring frequently, until the vegetables are crisp-tender, about 5 minutes.

3. Add the garlic and cook, stirring constantly, until the garlic is fragrant, about 30 seconds.

4. In a small bowl, whisk together the coconut aminos, vinegar, and arrowroot.

5. Add it to the cooked vegetables and cook, stirring constantly, until the sauce simmers and thickens, about 4 minutes.

6. Serve the stir-fry over the Cauliflower "Rice."

PER SERVING Calories: 177; Total Fat: 7g; Saturated Fat: 6g; Cholesterol: 0mg; Carbohydrates: 26g; Fiber: 6g; Protein: 4g

VEGGIE "RICE" BOWL

Serves 4 / Prep time: 10 minutes / Cook time: 15 minutes

WEEK 4

Arrowroot powder thickens the sauce in this stir-fry. You should be able to find it with other specialty flours in the baking aisle at the grocery store. Arrowroot is a starch obtained from the rhizomes of different tropical plants.

NIGHTSHADE-
FREE

NUT-FREE

VEGAN

QUICK &
EASY

2 tablespoons coconut oil

½ onion, thinly sliced

2 cups broccoli florets

2 cups baby spinach

2 garlic cloves, minced

2 tablespoons coconut aminos

1 tablespoon rice vinegar

1 teaspoon Asian fish sauce

½ teaspoon fresh grated ginger

2 tablespoons arrowroot powder

¼ cup chopped fresh cilantro

1 recipe Cauliflower "Rice" (page 231)

2 scallions, thinly sliced

1. In a large sauté pan over medium-high heat, heat the coconut oil until it shimmers. Add the onion and cook, stirring occasionally, until it is soft, about 5 minutes.

2. Add the broccoli and spinach and cook, stirring frequently, until the vegetables begin to soften, about 5 minutes more.

3. Add the garlic and cook, stirring constantly, until it is fragrant, about 30 seconds.

4. In a small bowl, whisk together the coconut aminos, rice vinegar, fish sauce, ginger, arrowroot powder, and cilantro. Pour the mixture into the pan with the vegetables, bring it to a simmer, and cook on medium, stirring frequently, for 5 more minutes.

5. Toss the vegetables with the Cauliflower "Rice," garnish with the sliced scallions, and serve.

Ingredient tip: Asian fish sauce is made from fermented anchovies and can be found at Asian markets and gourmet grocers, or can be purchased online. It is intensely flavored but does not add a fishy flavor to foods. Instead it adds umami—a deep, savory taste.

PER SERVING Calories: 163; Total Fat: 10g; Saturated Fat: 6g; Cholesterol: 0mg; Carbohydrates: 17g; Fiber: 5g; Protein: 5g

ZUCCHINI "PASTA" WITH WALNUT AND SPINACH PESTO

Serves 4 / Prep time: 10 minutes / Cook time: 7 minutes

Zucchini takes the place of pasta in this easy recipe. In the pesto, feel free to replace the walnuts with another tree nut, such as almonds. You may also choose to use the more classic pesto nut: pignolis—also called pine nuts.

NIGHTSHADE-
FREE

VEGAN

FOR THE "PASTA"

2 tablespoons coconut oil

2 medium zucchini, cut into spaghetti strips

2 garlic cloves, minced

¼ cup water

½ teaspoon sea salt

¼ teaspoon freshly ground black pepper

FOR THE PESTO

3 garlic cloves

1 (9-ounce) package baby spinach leaves

6 large basil leaves

½ cup walnuts

¼ cup extra-virgin olive oil

½ teaspoon sea salt

¼ teaspoon freshly ground black pepper

TO MAKE THE "PASTA"

1. In a large sauté pan over medium-high heat, heat the coconut oil until it shimmers.

2. Add the zucchini strips and cook them, stirring constantly, for 1 minute.

3. Add the garlic and cook, stirring constantly, until it is fragrant, about 30 seconds.

4. Add the water, salt, and pepper, and cook, stirring occasionally, until the zucchini is soft, about 6 minutes.

5. Drain the zucchini in a colander.

TO MAKE THE PESTO

1. In the bowl of a food processor fitted with a chopping blade, process the garlic, spinach, basil, walnuts, olive oil, salt, and pepper until all the ingredients are finely chopped, 30 seconds to 1 minute.

2. Toss the pesto with the hot zucchini, and serve immediately.

Time-saving tip: To turn the zucchini into noodles, you can use a kitchen gadget called a spiralizer. If you don't have one, don't worry. Use a vegetable peeler to cut long strips from the zucchini, and then cut those strips into thin "noodles" with a sharp knife.

PER SERVING Calories: 301; Total Fat: 30g; Saturated Fat: 8g; Cholesterol: 0mg; Carbohydrates: 9g; Fiber: 4g; Protein: 7g

STUFFED ZUCCHINI

Serves 4 / Prep time: 10 minutes / Cook time: 60 minutes

These zucchini are stuffed with a flavorful mix of chopped nuts, vegetables, and herbs, which makes for a satisfying, nutritious meal. You can bake the zucchini ahead of time and store them in the refrigerator. Then, stuff them and finish them in the oven for a quick weeknight meal.

VEGETARIAN

4 medium zucchini

4 tablespoons coconut oil, melted, divided

1 onion, minced

1 green bell pepper, seeded and chopped

1 jalapeño pepper, seeded and chopped

8 ounces cremini mushrooms, very finely chopped

4 garlic cloves, minced

1 teaspoon dried thyme

1 teaspoon dried rosemary

1 cup Slow Cooker Vegetable Broth (page 227)

2 cups almond flour

1 egg, beaten

1 teaspoon sea salt

¼ teaspoon freshly ground black pepper

¼ teaspoon red pepper flakes

1. Preheat the oven to 375°F.

2. Cut a strip off the top of the zucchini. Using a spoon, scoop out the zucchini pulp and leave the shell. Set aside the zucchini pulp for another use, and put the shells on a baking sheet, cut-side up.

3. Drizzle the zucchini with 2 tablespoons of coconut oil, and bake for 20 minutes.

4. While the zucchini bake, heat the remaining 2 tablespoons of coconut oil in a large pot over medium-high heat.

5. Add the onion and cook, stirring occasionally, until it is soft, about 5 minutes.

6. Add the green pepper and jalapeño and cook until they are soft, another 5 minutes.

7. Add the mushrooms and cook, stirring occasionally, until the mushrooms release their liquid and begin to brown, 5 minutes more.

8. Add the garlic and cook, stirring constantly, until it is fragrant, about 30 seconds.

9. Add the thyme, rosemary, and Slow Cooker Vegetable Broth. Simmer for 5 more minutes, and remove from the heat.

10. Stir in the almond flour, egg, salt, pepper, and red pepper flakes, mixing to combine.

11. Scoop the mixture into the pre-baked zucchini shells. Return them to the oven and bake for 30 to 40 minutes more, until the filling is browned, and serve.

PER SERVING Calories: 286; Total Fat: 22g; Saturated Fat: 13g; Cholesterol: 41mg; Carbohydrates: 17g; Fiber: 7g; Protein: 10g

SHIITAKE AND ZUCCHINI HASH WITH POACHED EGGS

Serves 4 / Prep time: 10 minutes / Cook time: 20 minutes

WEEK 4

NIGHTSHADE-FREE

NUT-FREE

VEGETARIAN

QUICK & EASY

Shiitake mushrooms add umami—deep savoriness—to this delicious vegetable hash. Use fresh herbs in the hash for a very bright flavor. Serve the dish with the poached eggs spooned on top of the hash so the yolks will run through the vegetables like a sauce.

FOR THE HASH

2 tablespoons coconut oil

8 ounces shiitake mushrooms, sliced

½ onion, minced

1 medium zucchini, cut into ½-inch dice

½ teaspoon sea salt

¼ teaspoon freshly ground black pepper

2 garlic cloves, minced

1 tablespoon chopped fresh thyme

FOR THE EGGS

1 tablespoon vinegar

4 eggs

Sea salt

Freshly ground black pepper

1 tablespoon chopped fresh chives

TO MAKE THE HASH

1. In a large sauté pan over medium-high heat, heat the coconut oil until it shimmers.

2. Add the mushrooms, onion, zucchini, sea salt, and black pepper. Cook over medium-high heat, without stirring, until the mushrooms release their liquid and the liquid evaporates, 3 to 4 minutes.

3. Reduce the heat to low and continue to cook, stirring occasionally, until the vegetables are soft and browned, about 10 minutes more.

4. Add the garlic and thyme and cook, stirring constantly, until they are fragrant, about 30 seconds.

TO MAKE THE EGGS

1. Fill a large saucepan half full with water and add the vinegar. Over medium heat, bring the water to a simmer.

2. Using a spoon, stir to create a whirlpool in the simmering water. Crack the eggs and slip them into the whirlpool, one at a time. Cook for 5 minutes.

3. Using a slotted spoon, remove the eggs and allow them to drain. Place the eggs on top of the hash.

4. Sprinkle with sea salt, black pepper, and chopped chives and serve.

PER SERVING Calories: 171; Total Fat: 12g; Saturated Fat: 7g; Cholesterol: 164mg; Carbohydrates: 12g; Fiber: 2g; Protein: 7g

SPAGHETTI SQUASH MARINARA

Serves 4 / Prep time: 10 minutes / Cook time: 60 minutes

While spaghetti squash takes about an hour to cook, it's all passive time. You can put your marinara sauce together in the last twenty minutes of cooking the squash. Marinara uses an array of fresh vegetables that are available in the summer.

NUT-FREE

VEGAN

1 spaghetti squash
2 tablespoons coconut oil
1 onion, minced
1 red bell pepper, seeded and minced
6 garlic cloves, minced
2 tablespoons tomato paste
3 carrots, peeled and diced
2 (15-ounce) cans crushed tomatoes and their juice
1 teaspoon dried oregano
⅛ teaspoon red pepper flakes
1 teaspoon sea salt
¼ teaspoon freshly ground black pepper
2 tablespoons chopped fresh basil
¼ cup chopped fresh Italian parsley

1. Preheat the oven to 375°F.
2. Put the spaghetti squash on a baking sheet.
3. Bake the spaghetti squash for 1 hour, until you can easily pierce it with a knife.
4. Halve the squash lengthwise. Using a fork, scrape out the flesh into "noodles."
5. While the squash is baking, in a large pot, heat the coconut oil over medium-high heat until it shimmers. Add the onion and cook, stirring occasionally, until it is soft and starts to brown, 5 to 7 minutes.
6. Add the red bell pepper and cook, stirring occasionally, until it softens, about 5 minutes more.

7. Add the garlic and cook, stirring constantly, until it is fragrant, about 30 seconds.

8. Add the tomato paste and cook, stirring constantly, for 2 minutes more.

9. Add the carrots, crushed tomatoes and their juice, oregano, pepper flakes, salt, and pepper. Bring to a simmer, stirring frequently; then reduce the heat to medium. Simmer until the carrots are soft, about 10 minutes more.

10. Remove the pot from the heat and stir in the basil and parsley. Serve spooned over the spaghetti squash.

PER SERVING Calories: 199; Total Fat: 7g; Saturated Fat: 6g; Cholesterol: 0mg; Carbohydrates: 30g; Fiber: 10g; Protein: 7g

SPAGHETTI SQUASH WITH THREE-PEPPER SAUCE

Serves 4 / Prep time: 10 minutes / Cook time: 60 minutes

Red, yellow, and orange bell peppers combine with garlic and onions to make a sweet yet slightly spicy sauce, providing a flavorful "pasta" dish. You can also use the sauce to top zucchini "pasta," or as a delicious topping for steamed vegetables.

NUT-FREE

VEGAN

1 spaghetti squash

2 tablespoons coconut oil

1 onion, minced

1 red bell pepper, seeded and chopped

1 yellow bell pepper, seeded and chopped

1 orange bell pepper, seeded and chopped

6 garlic cloves, minced

1 cup Slow Cooker Vegetable Broth (page 227)

1 teaspoon sea salt

¼ teaspoon freshly ground black pepper

⅛ teaspoon red pepper flakes

1. Preheat the oven to 375°F.

2. Put the spaghetti squash on a baking sheet and bake for 1 hour, until you can easily pierce it with a knife.

3. Halve the squash lengthwise. Using a fork, scrape out the flesh into "noodles."

4. While the squash is baking, in a large pot over medium-high heat, heat the coconut oil until it shimmers. Add the onion and cook, stirring occasionally, until it is soft and starts to brown, 5 to 7 minutes.

5. Add the red, yellow, and orange peppers and cook, stirring occasionally, until they soften, about 5 minutes more.

6. Add the garlic and cook, stirring constantly, until it is fragrant, about 30 seconds.

7. Add the Slow Cooker Vegetable Broth, salt, pepper, and red pepper flakes. Reduce the heat to medium-low and cover the pot. Simmer until the peppers are soft, about 10 minutes.

8. Pour the sauce into a food processor or blender. Blend until the sauce is smooth, about 30 seconds.

9. Spoon the warm sauce over the spaghetti squash and serve.

Cooking tip: When blending hot food in a food processor or blender, safety is important. Place a folded towel over the top of the lid, and put your hand on top of it to hold it in place. Then, every few seconds, turn off the blender and allow the steam to escape through the lid of the blender or the chute of the food processor to avoid pressure buildup.

PER SERVING Calories: 145; Total Fat: 8g; Saturated Fat: 6g; Cholesterol: 0mg; Carbohydrates: 17g; Fiber: 3g; Protein: 3g

ASIAN PORTOBELLO LETTUCE WRAPS WITH ALMOND SAUCE

Serves 6 / Prep time: 10 minutes / Cook time: 20 minutes

Meaty portobello mushrooms combine with an Asian flavor profile and creamy almond butter sauce for these delicious lettuce wraps. You can use butter lettuce leaves or romaine lettuce leaves, both of which hold up well to the mushrooms. Use the large outer leaves to make the lettuce wraps.

NIGHTSHADE-FREE

VEGAN

QUICK & EASY

FOR THE ALMOND SAUCE

½ cup almond butter

Juice of 2 limes

½ cup coconut aminos

½ jalapeño pepper, seeded and finely minced

½ teaspoon fresh grated ginger

½ cup coconut milk

½ teaspoon Asian fish sauce

FOR THE LETTUCE WRAPS

2 tablespoons coconut oil

1 tablespoon fresh grated ginger

½ onion, sliced

4 portobello mushrooms, stemmed, cleaned, and cut into ¼-inch slices

3 garlic cloves, minced

1 tablespoon coconut aminos

½ teaspoon sea salt

¼ teaspoon freshly ground black pepper

2 tablespoons chopped fresh cilantro

12 large butter or romaine lettuce leaves

6 scallions, thinly sliced

TO MAKE THE ALMOND SAUCE

1. In a food processor or blender, process the almond butter, lime juice, coconut aminos, jalapeño, ginger, coconut milk, and fish sauce until smooth.

2. Set aside for a few minutes to let the flavors blend.

TO MAKE THE LETTUCE WRAPS

1. In a large sauté pan, heat the coconut oil over medium-high heat until it shimmers. Add the ginger and onion and cook, stirring frequently, until they are soft, about 5 minutes.

2. Add the mushrooms and cook, stirring occasionally, until they are browned, about 7 minutes.

3. Add the garlic and cook, stirring constantly, until it is fragrant, about 30 seconds.

4. Add the coconut aminos, sea salt, and pepper, and cook for another 3 minutes, stirring frequently.

5. Remove the mushroom mixture from the heat, and stir in the cilantro.

6. Serve the mushrooms wrapped in lettuce leaves, topped with the scallions, and dipped in the almond sauce.

Cooking tip: To clean the portobello, remove the stems. Then use a spoon to scrape away all of the black gills. Finally, use a mushroom brush or a paper towel to wipe the mushrooms clean. Do not rinse the mushrooms, because they will soak up too much water.

PER SERVING Calories: 390; Total Fat: 37g; Saturated Fat: 20g; Cholesterol: 43mg; Carbohydrates: 10g; Fiber: 3g; Protein: 8g

HUEVOS RANCHEROS

Serves 4 / Prep time: 10 minutes / Cook time: 20 minutes

Typically, huevos rancheros are made with spicy black beans. However, since beans are out on your diet, this version pairs the eggs with a spicy veggie sauce made from peppers, chiles, and tomato sauce. Serve topped with creamy avocado to cool things down a little.

4 tablespoons coconut oil, divided
1 onion, chopped
½ green bell pepper, seeded and chopped
½ red bell pepper, seeded and chopped
1 jalapeño pepper, seeded and chopped
3 garlic cloves, minced
1 (14-ounce) can crushed tomatoes and their juice
¼ teaspoon ground cayenne pepper
1 teaspoon ground cumin
1 tablespoon chili powder
½ teaspoon sea salt, plus more for seasoning
¼ teaspoon freshly ground black pepper, plus more for seasoning
8 eggs
1 avocado, peeled, pitted, and sliced

1. In a large sauté pan over medium-high heat, heat 2 tablespoons of coconut oil until it shimmers. Add the onions, green and red peppers, and jalapeño, and cook, stirring occasionally, until the vegetables are soft, about 5 minutes.

2. Add the garlic and cook, stirring constantly, until it is fragrant, about 30 seconds.

3. Add the tomatoes and their juice, cayenne, cumin, chili powder, salt, and pepper. Reduce the heat to medium and simmer, stirring occasionally, for about 5 minutes more.

4. While the sauce finishes cooking, heat the remaining 2 tablespoons coconut oil over medium heat in a large, nonstick fry pan.

5. Crack the eggs into the oil and cook until the whites are opaque, about 4 minutes.

6. Season the eggs with salt and pepper, and flip them. Turn off the heat, and allow them to sit another 60 seconds.

7. Put the eggs on 4 plates, top each with an equal amount of the tomato sauce and sliced avocado, and serve.

PER SERVING Calories: 432; Total Fat: 33g; Saturated Fat: 17g; Cholesterol: 327mg; Carbohydrates: 22g; Fiber: 10g; Protein: 16g

ASPARAGUS CRUSTLESS QUICHE

Serves 4 / Prep time: 10 minutes / Cook time: 45 minutes

WEEK 1

You can make this quiche ahead of time and store it in a tightly sealed container. Then warm it up in the microwave when you're ready to eat. Asparagus is a delicious spring vegetable. Find the stalks that are thin and tender for best results.

NIGHTSHADE-
FREE

NUT-FREE

VEGETARIAN

MAKE-AHEAD

Coconut oil, for greasing
6 eggs, beaten
½ cup coconut milk
1 tablespoon Dijon mustard
1 teaspoon onion powder
1 teaspoon garlic powder
½ teaspoon sea salt
¼ teaspoon freshly ground black pepper
2 cups asparagus, cut into 1-inch pieces

1. Preheat the oven to 350°F.
2. Grease a 9-inch pie plate with coconut oil.
3. In a large bowl, whisk together the eggs, coconut milk, mustard, onion powder, garlic powder, salt, and pepper until well combined.
4. Fold in the asparagus.
5. Pour the mixture into the prepared pie plate.
6. Bake the quiche until it sets, about 45 minutes.
7. Allow the quiche to rest for 10 minutes before slicing and serving.

Ingredient tip: To prepare the asparagus, hold the stalk at both ends and bend it slightly. It will snap at the place where the stalk begins to get tender. Discard the tough bottom of the stalk.

PER SERVING Calories: 184; Total Fat: 14g; Saturated Fat: 8g; Cholesterol: 246mg; Carbohydrates: 6g; Fiber: 2g; Protein: 11g

PUMPKIN COCONUT SOUP

Serves 4 / Prep time: 10 minutes / Cook time: 30 minutes

WEEK 2

The perfect fall recipe, this creamy pumpkin soup is flavorful and satisfying. Along with pumpkin, the soup has the warm scent of sage—the quintessential fall herb. Enjoy a bowl of this hearty soup for lunch or dinner. It also freezes well.

NIGHTSHADE-FREE

NUT-FREE

VEGAN

MAKE-AHEAD

2 tablespoons coconut oil

1 onion, chopped

2 carrots, peeled and chopped

3 cups Slow Cooker Vegetable Broth (page 227)

1 (14-ounce) can pumpkin purée

3 sage leaves

1 (14-ounce) can coconut milk

½ teaspoon sea salt

¼ teaspoon freshly ground black pepper

1. In a large pot over medium-high heat, heat the coconut oil until it shimmers.

2. Add the onion and cook, stirring occasionally, until it softens, about 5 minutes.

3. Add the carrots and cook, stirring occasionally, until the carrots begin to soften, about 5 minutes more.

4. Add the Slow Cooker Vegetable Broth, pumpkin purée, sage leaves, coconut milk, salt, and pepper. Bring the soup to a simmer; then reduce the heat to medium and simmer for 20 minutes.

5. Remove the sage leaves from the soup. Purée the soup in the food processor or blender until it is smooth, about 30 seconds, and serve.

Substitution tip: You can also make this soup with any winter squash purée in place of the pumpkin.

PER SERVING Calories: 429; Total Fat: 37g; Saturated Fat: 32g; Cholesterol: 0mg; Carbohydrates: 23g; Fiber: 8g; Protein: 8g

SWEET POTATO CURRY

Serves 4 / Prep time: 15 minutes / Cook time: 45 minutes

WEEK 3

This warm curry is a great way to unwind after a long day. Fragrant with curry spices and subtly layered with flavor, it is a satisfying and delicious meal. You can use any type of sweet potato or yam for this recipe.

NIGHTSHADE-
FREE

NUT-FREE

VEGAN

4 tablespoons coconut oil, divided

2 tablespoons curry powder

1 (14-ounce) can coconut milk

1 onion, chopped

8 ounces shiitake mushrooms, sliced

4 garlic cloves, minced

4 sweet potatoes, cut into ½-inch cubes

1 cup Slow Cooker Vegetable Broth (page 227)

1 teaspoon sea salt

¼ teaspoon freshly ground black pepper

1. In a small pot over medium-high heat, heat 2 tablespoons of coconut oil until it shimmers.

2. Add the curry powder and cook, stirring constantly, until it is fragrant, about 1 minute.

3. Add the coconut milk, and reduce the heat to medium. Simmer while you prepare the rest of the meal.

4. In a large pot, heat the remaining 2 tablespoons of coconut oil over medium-high heat until it shimmers. Add the onion and cook, stirring occasionally, until it softens, about 5 minutes.

5. Add the mushrooms and cook, stirring occasionally, until they brown, about 5 minutes more.

6. Add the garlic and cook, stirring constantly, until it is fragrant, about 30 seconds.

7. Add the curry-coconut milk mixture, sweet potatoes, Slow Cooker Vegetable Broth, salt, and pepper to the pot. Bring to a simmer, and reduce the heat to medium-low.

8. Simmer until the potatoes are soft, about 20 minutes, and serve.

PER SERVING Calories: 485; Total Fat: 29g; Saturated Fat: 25g; Cholesterol: 0mg; Carbohydrates: 55g; Fiber: 10g; Protein: 6g

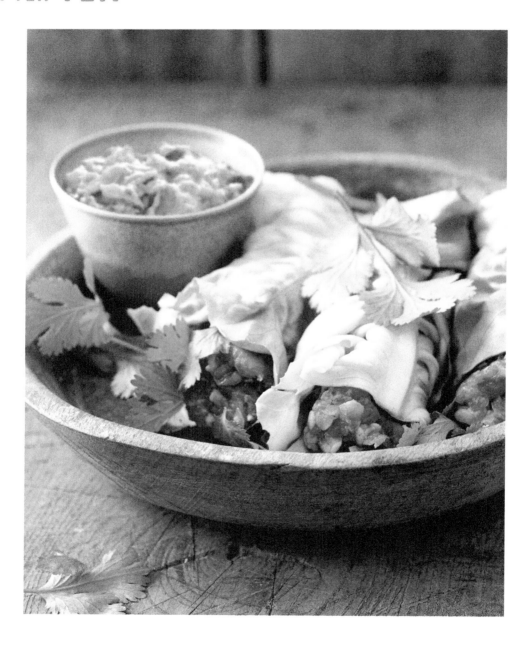

CHAPTER TEN

FISH AND SEAFOOD DINNERS

SEARED SEA SCALLOPS WITH CITRUS SPINACH

Serves 4 / Prep time: 10 minutes / Cook time: 20 minutes

3-DAY CLEANSE / WEEK 4

NIGHTSHADE-FREE

NUT-FREE

QUICK & EASY

The orange flavor in the spinach works well with the sweetness of sea scallops. Choose large scallops that have an opalescent sheen. If possible, buy fresh and not previously frozen scallops. If you must buy frozen, choose flash-frozen scallops and thaw them in the bag in a sink full of cold water.

1 pound sea scallops
Sea salt
Freshly ground black pepper
4 tablespoons animal fat, such as lard or duck fat, divided
2 garlic cloves, minced
1 (9-ounce) package baby spinach
Juice and zest of 1 orange

1. In a colander, rinse the scallops and pat them dry with a paper towel. Using a sharp knife, remove the tendons along the sides of the scallops. Season the scallops with salt and pepper.

2. In a large sauté pan over medium-high heat, heat 2 tablespoons of fat until it shimmers. Add the scallops in a single layer and cook without moving them until they caramelize on the bottom, about 2 minutes. Flip the scallops and cook on the other side, 2 to 3 more minutes, until the scallops are browned on both sides.

3. Remove the scallops from the pan and set them aside on a plate, tented with foil.

4. Add the remaining 2 tablespoons of fat to the pan. Add the garlic and cook, stirring constantly, for 30 seconds.

5. Add the spinach and cook, stirring constantly, until it begins to wilt. Add the orange juice and orange zest. Cook for another 2 to 3 minutes, until the spinach is cooked through. Season with salt and pepper.

6. Serve the scallops on top of the spinach.

Ingredient tip: Not all sea scallops have the tendon on the side. If the scallop is round and smooth, there is nothing to remove. If there is a small band attached along the side of the scallop, you will need to remove it because the tendon is tough.

PER SERVING Calories: 251; Total Fat: 2g; Saturated Fat: 0g; Cholesterol: 75mg; Carbohydrates: 15g; Fiber: 3g; Protein: 43g

SHRIMP MOJO WITH MUSHROOMS

Serves 4 / Prep time: 10 minutes / Cook time: 90 minutes

WEEK 3

Garlic mojo is easy to make and doesn't require a lot of hands-on time. It just takes time to cook in the oven. You can make the garlic mojo ahead of time, and then measure some out when it comes time to cook the shrimp. The mojo will keep in the refrigerator for about 2 months.

NIGHTSHADE-
FREE

NUT-FREE

MAKE-AHEAD

FOR THE MOJO

Cloves from 2 heads of garlic, peeled and smashed

1 cup extra-virgin olive oil

Juice of 1 lime

½ teaspoon sea salt

FOR THE SHRIMP AND MUSHROOMS

¼ cup garlic mojo, with pieces of garlic in it

1 pound shrimp (26 to 30 count), peeled, deveined, and tails removed

1 onion, chopped

8 ounces cremini mushrooms, quartered

Juice of 1 lime

½ teaspoon sea salt

¼ teaspoon freshly ground black pepper

1 avocado, peeled, pitted, and sliced

4 lime wedges

TO MAKE THE MOJO

1. Preheat the oven to 325°F.

2. In an ovenproof glass bread pan, mix the garlic and olive oil. Roast until the garlic softens, about 50 minutes.

3. Squeeze the lime juice into the mojo, and add the salt. Continue cooking it for 20 more minutes then cool completely.

4. Store it in the refrigerator, tightly sealed in a glass Mason jar.

TO MAKE THE SHRIMP AND MUSHROOMS

1. In a large sauté pan over medium-high heat, heat the mojo.
2. Add the shrimp and onions, and cook, stirring frequently, until it is pink, about 4 minutes. Using a slotted spoon, remove the shrimp from the pan and set aside on a platter tented with foil.
3. Add the mushrooms to the same pan and cook, stirring frequently, until they are browned and soft, about 5 minutes.
4. Add the lime juice, salt, pepper, cooked shrimp, and any juices that have collected on the platter. Cook until the shrimp are warmed through, 3 to 4 minutes.
5. Serve the shrimp in a bowl garnished with avocado slices and lime wedges.

Cooking tip: To smash the garlic, lay each clove on its side and put the flat side of a chef's knife over the garlic. Then, using your fist, smash the flat of the knife, crushing the garlic beneath.

PER SERVING Calories: 389; Total Fat: 25g; Saturated Fat: 5g; Cholesterol: 239mg; Carbohydrates: 15g; Fiber: 5g; Protein: 30g

CRAB CAKES WITH LEMON-LIME MAYONNAISE

Serves 4 / Prep time: 10 minutes / Cook time: 5 minutes

These rich crab cakes go well with the Apple and Ginger Slaw on page 133 or some steamed green beans. Top them with this rich lemon-lime sauce that perfectly complements the richness of the crab cake. You can find lump crab meat in the seafood section at your local grocery store.

FOR THE LEMON-LIME MAYONNAISE

1 cup Homemade Mayonnaise (page 229)

Juice and zest of ½ lemon

Juice and zest of 1 lime

FOR THE CRAB CAKES

1 pound lump crab meat, picked over and drained

4 scallions, thinly sliced

½ teaspoon onion powder

½ teaspoon garlic powder

1 tablespoon chopped fresh chives

⅔ cups almond flour, divided

Juice of ½ lemon

1 large egg, beaten

½ cup Homemade Mayonnaise (page 229)

1 tablespoon Dijon mustard

½ teaspoon sea salt

¼ teaspoon freshly ground black pepper

2 tablespoons animal fat, such as duck fat or lard

TO MAKE THE LEMON-LIME MAYONNAISE

1. In a small bowl, whisk together the Homemade Mayonnaise, lemon juice, lemon zest, lime juice, and lime zest.

2. Set aside to let the flavors blend.

TO MAKE THE CRAB CAKES

1. In a large bowl, stir together the crab meat, scallions, onion powder, garlic powder, chives, and ⅓ cup of almond flour.

2. In a small bowl, whisk together the lemon juice, egg, Homemade Mayonnaise, mustard, salt, and pepper. Pour the mayonnaise mixture into the crab mixture, and carefully fold it with a rubber spatula to combine.

3. Form the mixture into 8 crab cakes, and use the remaining ⅓ cup of almond flour to coat each cake.

4. In a large sauté pan over medium-high heat, heat the fat.

5. Working in 2 batches, cook the crab cakes until they are golden on both sides, about 3 minutes per side. Blot on paper towels before serving.

6. Serve the crab cakes with the lemon-lime mayonnaise spooned over the top.

Ingredient tip: Check through all the lump crab meat, and remove any shell pieces before making the crab cakes.

PER SERVING Calories: 587; Total Fat: 52g; Saturated Fat: 8g; Cholesterol: 140mg; Carbohydrates: 30g; Fiber: 3g; Protein: 22g

SHRIMP SCAMPI WITH ZUCCHINI NOODLES

Serves 4 / Prep time: 10 minutes / Cook time: 20 minutes

WEEK 2

NIGHTSHADE-
FREE

NUT-FREE

QUICK &
EASY

With garlic, lemon, and parsley, this shrimp dish packs a lot of Italian flavor. If possible, use fresh shrimp. If you can't find fresh shrimp, then wild-caught frozen shrimp will work. For best results, use shrimp that is about 26 to 30 count per pound or larger.

2 tablespoons animal fat, such as lard or duck fat
1 pound shrimp, peeled, deveined, and tails removed
5 garlic cloves, minced
Juice and zest of 1 lemon
¼ cup Slow Cooker Bone Broth (page 226)
¼ cup chopped fresh Italian parsley
½ teaspoon sea salt
¼ teaspoon freshly ground black pepper
1 recipe Zucchini "Spaghetti" (page 232)

1. In a large sauté pan over medium-high heat, heat the fat until it shimmers. Add the shrimp and cook, stirring frequently, until they turn pink.

2. Add the garlic and cook, stirring constantly, until it is fragrant, about 30 seconds.

3. Add the lemon juice, lemon zest, Slow Cooker Bone Broth, parsley, salt, and pepper. Bring to a simmer, and remove from the heat.

4. Toss the shrimp with the hot Zucchini "Spaghetti" and serve.

Ingredient tip: Before cooking fresh shrimp, you'll need to clean it. Under running water, use a sharp paring knife to remove the shell and tail. Then make a shallow slit along the back of the shrimp, and use the tip of the knife to remove the vein.

PER SERVING Calories: 216; Total Fat: 9g; Saturated Fat: 3g; Cholesterol: 245mg; Carbohydrates: 6g; Fiber: 1g; Protein: 27g

GINGER SALMON WITH SWEET POTATO MASH

Serves 4 / Prep time: 20 minutes / Cook time: 25 minutes

WEEK 4

The marinade of coconut aminos and ginger imparts tremendous flavor to this tasty fish. Salmon is extremely healthy because it contains high amounts of anti-inflammatory omega-3 fatty acids. Use only wild-caught salmon, as farm-raised salmon has high levels of chemicals called PCBs.

¼ cup coconut aminos

¼ cup extra-virgin olive oil

1 tablespoon fresh grated ginger

4 (4-ounce) salmon fillets

2 sweet potatoes, peeled and cut into ½-inch pieces

¼ cup unsweetened coconut milk

½ teaspoon sea salt

¼ teaspoon freshly ground black pepper

FODMAP-FREE

NIGHTSHADE-FREE

NUT-FREE

1. In a small bowl, whisk together the coconut aminos, olive oil, and ginger. Pour the mixture into a shallow dish, and put the salmon, flesh-side down, in the marinade. Marinate for 20 minutes.

2. While the salmon marinates, put the potatoes in a large pot of water and bring to a boil. Boil the sweet potatoes until they are soft, about 20 minutes. In a colander, drain the potatoes.

3. Preheat the oven to 425°F.

4. When the salmon is done marinating, put it on a baking sheet and bake, skin-side down, until the flesh flakes easily, about 25 minutes.

5. Meanwhile, in a large bowl, using a potato masher, mash together the potatoes, coconut milk, salt, and pepper.

6. Serve the salmon with a mound of mashed sweet potatoes on the side.

PER SERVING Calories: 439; Total Fat: 24g; Saturated Fat: 6g; Cholesterol: 50mg; Carbohydrates: 34g; Fiber: 5g; Protein: 25g

STEAMER CLAMS IN LEMON-FENNEL BROTH

Serves 4 / Prep time: 10 minutes / Cook time: 15 minutes

WEEK 1 / WEEK 4

NIGHTSHADE-FREE

NUT-FREE

QUICK & EASY

The broth and vegetables that go with these clams are rich and flavorful. Pull the clams out of their shells to eat them, and drink the broth like a soup. Use small Manila or steamer clams for best results.

2 tablespoons animal fat, such as lard or duck fat

1 red onion, minced

1 fennel bulb, thinly sliced

3 garlic cloves, minced

2 pounds steamer clams, in shells

Juice of 2 lemons

Zest of 1 lemon

4 cups Slow Cooker Bone Broth (page 226)

1 teaspoon sea salt

¼ teaspoon freshly ground black pepper

1 tablespoon chopped fresh tarragon

1 tablespoon chopped fennel fronds

1. In a large pot over medium-high heat, heat the animal fat until it shimmers. Add the onion and fennel and cook, stirring frequently, until the vegetables are soft, about 6 minutes.

2. Add the garlic and cook, stirring constantly, until it is fragrant, about 30 seconds.

3. Add the clams, lemon juice, lemon zest, bone broth, salt, and pepper. Cook, covered, until the clams open, about 10 minutes.

4. Remove from the heat, and stir in the tarragon. Serve in bowls, garnished with the chopped fennel fronds.

Ingredient tip: Any clams that don't open should be discarded because they may be spoiled. Pick over the clams before serving to ensure you've removed all unopened clams.

PER SERVING Calories: 243; Total Fat: 9g; Saturated Fat: 3g; Cholesterol: 6mg; Carbohydrates: 34g; Fiber: 3g; Protein: 8g

HALIBUT WITH BLACKBERRY SAUCE AND ASPARAGUS

Serves 4 / Prep time: 10 minutes / Cook time: 15 minutes

WEEK 2

NIGHTSHADE-FREE

NUT-FREE

QUICK & EASY

Juicy blackberries make a wonderful sweet-tart sauce that pairs well with sweet, mild halibut. You can find blackberries in late summer, so it's a great time to make this light, summery dish. Sauté the asparagus in animal fat with a little bit of salt and pepper for a simple side dish.

FOR THE BLACKBERRY SAUCE

2 tablespoons coconut oil

1 shallot, finely chopped

2 garlic cloves, minced

1 cup blackberries, mashed

¼ cup balsamic vinegar

½ teaspoon chopped fresh thyme

½ teaspoon sea salt

¼ teaspoon freshly ground black pepper

FOR THE ASPARAGUS

2 tablespoons animal fat

1 bunch asparagus, tough ends trimmed

Sea salt

Freshly ground black pepper

FOR THE HALIBUT

4 (4-ounce) halibut fillets

Sea salt

Freshly ground black pepper

TO MAKE THE BLACKBERRY SAUCE

1. In a large sauté pan over medium-high heat, heat the coconut oil until it shimmers. Add the shallots and cook, stirring frequently, until they are soft, about 4 minutes.

2. Add the garlic and cook, stirring constantly, until it is fragrant, about 30 seconds.

3. Add the blackberries, vinegar, thyme, salt, and pepper. Bring to a simmer, and reduce the heat to medium-low.

4. Simmer until the sauce reduces by half, about 10 minutes.

TO MAKE THE ASPARAGUS

1. In a large sauté pan over medium-high heat, heat the animal fat until it shimmers.

2. Add the asparagus and cook, stirring frequently, until it is tender, about 5 minutes.

3. Season with salt and pepper.

TO MAKE THE HALIBUT

1. Preheat the broiler to high.

2. Season the halibut with salt and pepper, and put it in a broiler pan.

3. Broil the halibut for 5 minutes. Turn the halibut and broil for another 3 minutes, until the fish is opaque.

4. Serve the fish with the blackberry sauce spooned over the top and the asparagus on the side.

PER SERVING Calories: 433; Total Fat: 19g; Saturated Fat: 9g; Cholesterol: 89mg; Carbohydrates: 7g; Fiber: 3g; Protein: 56g

COD WITH PEACH SALSA AND COCONUT CAULIFLOWER "RICE"

Serves 4 / Prep time: 15 minutes / Cook time: 15 minutes

WEEK 1

A summery, spicy salsa makes this cod delicious. Coconut cauliflower "rice" adds tropical flair for a composed, light dish that's perfect for a summer evening. The salsa is great on its own, as well. Use it as a dip for sliced jicama for a sweet, spicy, savory snack.

FOR THE COD

4 (4-ounce) cod fillets

Sea salt

Freshly ground black pepper

Juice of 1 lemon

FOR THE PEACH SALSA

3 peaches, pitted and chopped

½ red onion, diced

1 garlic clove, minced

2 tablespoons fresh cilantro, chopped

Juice of 1 lime

FOR THE COCONUT CAULIFLOWER "RICE"

2 tablespoons coconut oil

½ red onion, diced

2 garlic cloves, minced

½ cup coconut milk

1 recipe Cauliflower "Rice" (page 231)

4 lemon wedges

NIGHTSHADE-FREE

NUT-FREE

QUICK & EASY

TO MAKE THE COD

1. Preheat the broiler to high.

2. Adjust the oven rack so it is 3 to 4 inches below the broiler.

3. Season the cod with salt and pepper, put it on a broiling pan, and squeeze the lemon juice over the top.

4. Broil the cod until it is flaky, about 10 minutes.

TO MAKE THE PEACH SALSA

1. In a small bowl, mix together the peaches, onion, garlic, cilantro, and lime juice.

2. Set aside to let the flavors blend.

TO MAKE THE COCONUT CAULIFLOWER "RICE"

1. In a large sauté pan over medium-high heat, heat the coconut oil until it shimmers.

2. Add the onion and cook, stirring occasionally, until it is soft, about 5 minutes.

3. Add the garlic and cook, stirring constantly, until it is fragrant, about 30 seconds.

4. Add the coconut milk and Cauliflower "Rice." Cook, stirring frequently, until the rice is warm and the coconut milk is absorbed a little, about 5 minutes more.

5. Divide the rice evenly among four plates. Place a cod fillet on each bed of rice, and spoon some salsa on top of the cod. Serve with a lemon wedge on the side.

PER SERVING Calories: 306; Total Fat: 15g; Saturated Fat: 12g; Cholesterol: 52mg; Carbohydrates: 16g; Fiber: 4g; Protein: 29g

FISH TACOS

Serves 4 / Prep time: 20 minutes / Cook time: 10 minutes

WEEK 3

This fish taco filling, wrapped in lettuce leaves and served with guacamole, will add Latin flair to your next meal. While the recipe calls for halibut, you can use any flaky white fish, such as cod or mahimahi.

NIGHTSHADE-FREE

NUT-FREE

QUICK & EASY

Juice of 2 limes

¼ cup extra-virgin olive oil

¼ cup chopped fresh cilantro

3 garlic cloves, minced

16 ounces halibut fillets

8 large butter lettuce leaves

1 cup Guacamole (page 106)

1. In a small bowl, whisk together the lime juice, olive oil, cilantro, and garlic. Pour the marinade into a zipper bag, and add the halibut. Refrigerate and marinate for 20 minutes.

2. Preheat the broiler to high.

3. Adjust the rack to about 6 inches below the broiler.

4. Remove the halibut from the marinade, and pat it dry. Broil until the flesh flakes easily, about 10 minutes.

5. Cut the halibut into chunks. Serve wrapped in the lettuce leaves, topped with the Guacamole.

PER SERVING Calories: 476; Total Fat: 26g; Saturated Fat: 4g; Cholesterol: 82mg; Carbohydrates: 6g; Fiber: 3g; Protein: 55g

BAKED LEMON-DILL SALMON WITH CELERIAC PURÉE

Serves 4 / Prep time: 10 minutes / Cook time: 25 minutes

WEEK 1

Celeriac, also known as celery root, has a nutty flavor. When you purée it, the texture is similar to potatoes. To prepare it, use a potato peeler or a paring knife to cut away the tough, fibrous skin. Then, cut it into ½-inch chunks before boiling.

NIGHTSHADE-FREE

NUT-FREE

4 (4-ounce) salmon fillets
Sea salt
Freshly ground black pepper
8 dill sprigs
1 lemon, sliced
3 medium celeriac, peeled and cut into ½-inch pieces
8 garlic cloves, peeled
¼ cup Slow Cooker Bone Broth (page 226)
½ teaspoon sea salt
¼ teaspoon freshly ground black pepper
4 lemon wedges

1. Preheat the oven to 425°F.
2. Season the salmon with salt and pepper, and put it on a baking sheet, skin-side down. Lay 2 sprigs of dill and 1 or 2 lemon slices on top of each fillet. Bake the salmon until the flesh flakes easily, about 25 minutes.
3. Meanwhile, in a large pot filled with water, boil the celeriac and whole garlic cloves until the celeriac is soft, about 20 minutes.
4. In a colander, drain the celeriac and garlic. Put them in a blender or the bowl of a food processor with the broth, salt, and pepper. Purée until smooth, about 30 seconds.
5. Remove the lemon and dill from the salmon and serve on plates with the celeriac purée.

PER SERVING Calories: 211; Total Fat: 8g; Saturated Fat: 1g; Cholesterol: 50mg; Carbohydrates: 13g; Fiber: 2g; Protein: 25g

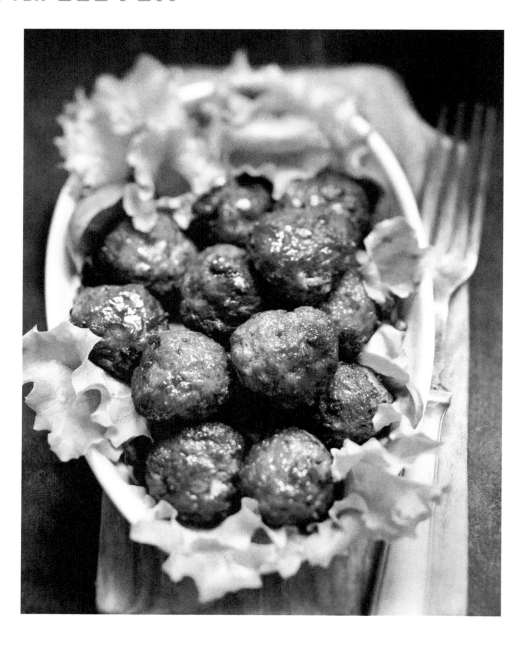

CHAPTER ELEVEN

MEAT AND POULTRY DINNERS

TURKEY PICCATA WITH LEMON ZUCCHINI

Serves 4 / Prep time: 10 minutes / Cook time: 20 minutes

3-DAY CLEANSE / WEEK 4

NIGHTSHADE-FREE

NUT-FREE

QUICK & EASY

Slice your turkey breast crosswise into ½-inch-thick slices. These slices cook quickly and combine well with the lemon and capers of the sauce. When combined with the herbed lemon zucchini, this quick and easy one-pan meal makes a flavorful weeknight dinner.

6 tablespoons animal fat, such as lard or duck fat, divided
1 medium zucchini, chopped
1 turkey breast, cut into ½-inch slices
Sea salt
Freshly ground black pepper
Juice of 3 lemons
1 shallot, finely chopped
2 tablespoons capers, rinsed
2 tablespoons chopped fresh Italian parsley

1. Preheat the oven to 200°F.
2. In a large sauté pan over medium-high heat, heat 2 tablespoons of fat until it shimmers. Add the zucchini and cook, stirring frequently, until it is soft, about 3 minutes.
3. Remove the zucchini from the pan, and set it aside on a plate.
4. Add the remaining 4 tablespoons of fat. Pound the turkey slices to ¼-inch thickness, and season with salt and pepper.
5. Cook the turkey slices in the hot fat until they are cooked, about 1 minute per side. Remove them from the fat and put them on the plate with the zucchini. Put the plate in the preheated oven to stay warm.

6. Add the lemon juice to the sauté pan, and add the shallot and capers. Bring to a simmer, and reduce the heat to medium-low. Simmer, stirring occasionally, until the liquid reduces by half.

7. Add the zucchini, turkey slices, and parsley to the pan.

8. Toss to coat the zucchini and turkey with the sauce and serve.

PER SERVING Calories: 308; Total Fat: 22g; Saturated Fat: 8g; Cholesterol: 67mg; Carbohydrates: 7g; Fiber: 1g; Protein: 20g

BACON-WRAPPED ROSEMARY CHICKEN LEGS WITH CARAMELIZED ONION GREEN BEANS

Serves 4 / Prep time: 20 minutes / Cook time: 60 minutes

WEEK 1 / WEEK 4

This is a recipe that stores well, so you can cook it over the weekend and have it as a great lunch or dinner for a busy weeknight. Simply put the cooked chicken in a tightly sealed zipper bag, and remove and reheat in the microwave later. The green beans reheat very well, too. Both the chicken and the beans also freeze well.

FOR THE CHICKEN

2 tablespoons chopped fresh rosemary

1 teaspoon sea salt

½ teaspoon freshly ground black pepper

8 chicken drumsticks

8 slices thin-cut bacon

FOR THE GREEN BEANS

2 slices bacon, chopped

1 onion, thinly sliced

8 ounces green beans, trimmed

¼ teaspoon sea salt

¼ teaspoon freshly ground black pepper

TO MAKE THE CHICKEN

1. Preheat the oven to 400°F.

2. In a small bowl, mix the rosemary, salt, and pepper. Sprinkle the chicken drumsticks with the mixture.

3. Wrap each piece of chicken with a piece of bacon.

4. Put the wrapped drumsticks in a 9-by-13-inch glass dish.

5. Bake the chicken for 1 hour.

NIGHTSHADE-FREE

NUT-FREE

MAKE-AHEAD

TO MAKE THE GREEN BEANS

1. While the chicken cooks, in a large sauté pan over medium-high heat, brown the bacon, about 5 minutes.

2. Using a slotted spoon, remove the bacon from the rendered fat and set it aside on a plate. Reduce the heat to medium-low, and add the onion to the fat. Cook, stirring occasionally, until the onion caramelizes, about 30 minutes.

3. While the onion cooks, bring a large pot of water to a boil over high heat. Blanch the green beans in the boiling water for 2 minutes. Remove the beans from the water, and plunge them into a bowl of ice water to stop cooking.

4. When the onions have caramelized, increase the heat to medium-high. Add the beans, reserved bacon, salt, and pepper to the sauté pan. Cook, stirring constantly, until the beans are heated through and crisp-tender, about 5 minutes more.

5. Serve with the chicken.

Cooking tip: To prepare the beans, trim off both ends. You can do this by lining up the ends of the beans and cutting several of them at a time with a sharp knife, repeating the process on the other side. You can also trim them one at a time. Depending on the length of the bean, you may also want to cut them in half.

PER SERVING Calories: 306; Total Fat: 15g; Saturated Fat: 5g; Cholesterol: 104mg; Carbohydrates: 8g; Fiber: 3g; Protein: 34g

STUFFED PORK TENDERLOIN WITH ROASTED ROOT VEGETABLES

Serves 4 / Prep time: 20 minutes, plus 4 hours to marinate /
Cook time: 30 minutes

WEEK 2

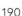
NIGHTSHADE-
FREE

NUT-FREE

MAKE-AHEAD

To stuff the pork tenderloin, you must first butterfly it. It is best to do so before you marinate the pork. Lay the pork loin on a cutting board and hold it in place with one hand, while the other hand holds the knife parallel to the board. Then cut lengthwise through the meat, stopping short of cutting it all the way through. You should be able to open the meat like a book into a flat piece before adding it to the marinade.

2 tablespoons Dijon mustard

¼ cup red wine vinegar

½ cup extra-virgin olive oil

3 garlic cloves, minced

1 teaspoon sea salt, divided

½ teaspoon freshly ground black pepper, divided

½ teaspoon dried sage

1 (1-pound) boneless pork loin, butterflied

1 sweet potato, cut into ½-inch cubes

2 carrots, peeled and cut into ½-inch rounds

1 parsnip, peeled and cut into ½-inch rounds

2 tablespoons animal fat, such as duck fat or lard, melted

4 ounces pancetta

2 cups baby spinach

1. In a large bowl, whisk together the mustard, vinegar, olive oil, garlic, 1/2 teaspoon of sea salt, 1/4 teaspoon of pepper, and the sage. Pour the marinade into a large resealable storage bag and add the butterflied tenderloin.

2. Marinate the meat for at least 4 hours in the refrigerator.

3. Preheat the oven to 425°F.

4. In a large bowl, toss together the sweet potato, carrots, parsnip, fat, and the remaining ½ teaspoon of salt and ¼ teaspoon of pepper. Arrange the vegetables in a large roasting pan, and cook in the oven for 15 minutes.

5. Meanwhile, remove the pork from the marinade and pat it dry. Put it on the counter, cut-side up. Line the pork with the slices of pancetta, then with the spinach.

6. Roll the roast up like a jelly roll, and tie it closed with butcher's twine.

7. Add the roast to the pan with the vegetables and continue cooking for another 30 minutes, until the pork and vegetables are done.

8. Allow the roast to rest for 10 minutes before serving.

PER SERVING Calories: 625; Total Fat: 42; Saturated Fat: 13; Cholesterol: 128mg; Carbohydrates: 17g; Fiber: 4g; Protein: 44g

ASIAN PORK MEATBALL LETTUCE WRAPS with DIPPING SAUCE

Serves 4 / Prep time: 20 minutes / Cook time: 30 minutes

With their Asian flavor, these meatballs make a tasty dinner for those nights when you really miss Asian takeout. As an added bonus, they are quick and easy to make. If you're not sensitive to nightshades and you want a little more heat, add some chili oil to the dipping sauce.

NIGHTSHADE-
FREE

NUT-FREE

MAKE-AHEAD

FOR THE DIPPING SAUCE

¼ cup coconut aminos

¼ cup rice vinegar

¼ teaspoon stevia

½ teaspoon fresh grated ginger

FOR THE MEATBALLS

1 pound ground pork

2 bunches scallions, thinly sliced

8 ounces shiitake mushrooms, finely chopped

¾ cup green cabbage, finely chopped

4 garlic cloves, minced

2 teaspoons fresh grated ginger

2 tablespoons chopped fresh cilantro

2 tablespoons coconut aminos

1 egg, beaten

½ teaspoon sea salt

¼ teaspoon freshly ground black pepper

8 butter lettuce leaves, from the outer part of the head

TO MAKE THE DIPPING SAUCE

1. In a small bowl, whisk together the coconut aminos, vinegar, stevia, and ginger.

2. Set aside to let the flavors blend.

TO MAKE THE MEATBALLS

1. Preheat the oven to 400°F.

2. Line a 9-by-13-inch baking sheet with parchment paper.

3. In a small bowl, mix the pork, scallions, mushrooms, cabbage, garlic, ginger, cilantro, coconut aminos, egg, salt, and pepper until well combined.

4. Roll the mixture into golf-ball-size balls and put them on the prepared baking sheet.

5. Bake until the meatballs are cooked, about 30 minutes.

6. Serve with the lettuce leaves for wrapping and the sauce for dipping.

Time-saving tip: To shorten the prep time, put the cabbage, mushrooms, garlic, ginger, and scallions in the bowl of a food processor fitted with a chopping blade. Pulse the food processor for 20 one-second pulses to finely chop the vegetables.

PER SERVING Calories: 250; Total Fat: 5g; Saturated Fat: 2g; Cholesterol: 124mg; Carbohydrates: 16g; Fiber: 3g; Protein: 35g

MEATLOAF MEATBALLS WITH BRUSSELS SPROUT HASH

Serves 4 / Prep time: 20 minutes / Cook time: 30 minutes

MAKE-AHEAD

Turning meatloaf mix into meatballs saves you about 30 minutes of cooking time over making a regular meatloaf. These meatballs taste just like little bites of meatloaf. While traditional meatloaf uses bread crumbs to bind them, these meatballs use almond meal instead.

FOR THE MEATBALLS

2 tablespoons coconut oil

½ onion, finely chopped

3 garlic cloves, minced

1 pound ground beef

½ cup almond meal

1 tablespoon Dijon mustard

1 teaspoon coconut aminos

1 teaspoon dried thyme

½ cup unsweetened almond milk

1 egg, beaten

1 tablespoon tomato paste

1 teaspoon sea salt

¼ teaspoon freshly ground black pepper

FOR THE HASH

2 tablespoons coconut oil

½ onion, finely diced

8 ounces Brussels sprouts, thinly sliced

2 garlic cloves, minced

2 tablespoons apple cider vinegar

¼ teaspoon stevia

½ teaspoon sea salt

¼ teaspoon freshly ground black pepper

TO MAKE THE MEATBALLS

1. Preheat the oven to 400°F.

2. Line a 9-by-13-inch baking sheet with parchment paper.

3. In a large sauté pan over medium-high heat, heat the coconut oil. Add the onion and cook, stirring occasionally, until it is soft, about 5 minutes.

4. Add the garlic and cook, stirring constantly, until it is fragrant, about 30 seconds more. Allow the onions and garlic to completely cool.

5. In a large bowl, mix the ground beef, almond meal, onions and garlic, mustard, coconut aminos, thyme, almond milk, egg, tomato paste, salt, and pepper until combined.

6. Roll the mixture into golf-ball-size balls and put them on the prepared baking sheet.

7. Bake until the meatballs are cooked through, about 30 minutes.

TO MAKE THE HASH

1. In a large sauté pan over medium-high heat, heat the coconut oil until it shimmers.

2. Add the onion and Brussels sprouts and cook, stirring frequently, until they are soft and start to brown, 6 to 7 minutes.

3. Add the garlic and cook, stirring constantly, until it is fragrant, about 30 seconds.

4. Add the apple cider vinegar, stevia, salt, and pepper, and simmer for another 3 minutes.

5. Serve with the meatballs.

PER SERVING Calories: 479; Total Fat: 30g; Saturated Fat: 15g; Cholesterol: 142mg; Carbohydrates: 14g; Fiber: 5g; Protein: 42g

SLOW COOKER COUNTRY-STYLE SPARE RIBS WITH APPLES AND FENNEL

Serves 6 / Prep time: 20 minutes / Cook time: 10 hours

WEEK 1

NIGHTSHADE-
FREE

NUT-FREE

MAKE-AHEAD

This is the perfect meal for a chilly fall evening. The combination of apples, fennel, and pork is a classic one. Using your slow cooker makes preparation very easy. Set it in the morning, and come home to a flavorful, warming dinner.

2 pounds country-style pork spare ribs

1 red onion, thinly sliced

2 sweet-tart apples, such as Honeycrisp, peeled, cored, and thinly sliced

1 fennel bulb, sliced

3 garlic cloves, minced

¼ cup apple cider vinegar

2 cups Slow Cooker Bone Broth (page 226)

1 teaspoon dried sage

1 teaspoon sea salt

½ teaspoon freshly ground black pepper

1. In the bowl of a large slow cooker, combine the ribs, onion, apples, fennel, garlic, vinegar, Slow Cooker Bone Broth, sage, salt, and pepper.

2. Cover and cook on low for 8 to 10 hours, until the pork is very tender.

Substitution tip: If you wish, you can toss in a head of thinly sliced cabbage to add even more veggies and fiber to this meal.

PER SERVING Calories: 362; Total Fat: 20g; Saturated Fat: 7g; Cholesterol: 93mg; Carbohydrates: 14g; Fiber: 3g; Protein: 32g

SLOW COOKER SLOPPY JOE BOWLS

Serves 4 / Prep time: 20 minutes / Cook time: 8 hours

Who says you need a bun for a sloppy Joe? These sloppy Joe bowls give you all the flavor without the gluten. To add crunch, top the sloppy Joes with your favorite coleslaw, or Jicama, Zucchini, and Avocado Slaw.

1 pound ground beef
1 onion, finely chopped
1 red bell pepper, finely chopped
1 green bell pepper, finely chopped
2 carrots, grated
1 celery rib, chopped
3 garlic cloves, minced
1 medium zucchini, chopped
2 tablespoons apple cider vinegar
1 (14-ounce) can crushed tomatoes, drained
½ teaspoon stevia
1 teaspoon sea salt
¼ teaspoon freshly ground black pepper
Jicama, Zucchini, and Avocado Slaw (page 135)

○
NUT-FREE

○
MAKE-AHEAD

1. In a large sauté pan over medium-high heat, heat the ground beef, crumbling it with a spatula as you cook, until it is browned, 8 to 10 minutes.

2. Add the ground beef to a slow cooker along with the onion, red and green bell peppers, carrots, celery, garlic, zucchini, vinegar, tomatoes, stevia, salt, and pepper.

3. Cook, covered, on low for 8 hours.

4. Serve in a bowl topped with the Jicama, Zucchini, and Avocado Slaw.

Substitution tip: If you'd like a "bun," make one out of portobello mushroom caps that have been cleaned and grilled.

PER SERVING Calories: 489; Total Fat: 18g; Saturated Fat: 5g; Cholesterol: 101mg; Carbohydrates: 42g; Fiber: 19g; Protein: 42g

SLOW COOKER HORSERADISH BRAISED BEEF RIBS WITH CAULIFLOWER MASH

Serves 8 / Prep time: 20 minutes / Cook time: 10 hours

WEEK 3

NIGHTSHADE-
FREE

NUT-FREE

To save time, you can prepare your cauliflower mash ahead of time and reheat it. If you do that, you'll spend about ten minutes in the morning preparing this delicious meal. It does take about ten extra minutes of prep time just before you serve it, but the results are well worth it.

3 pounds beef short ribs

8 ounces button mushrooms

4 carrots, chopped

1 onion, chopped

4 garlic cloves, minced

1 teaspoon dried thyme

1 tablespoon Dijon mustard

¼ cup red wine vinegar

2¼ cups Slow Cooker Bone Broth (page 226), or low-sodium
   canned broth, divided

1½ teaspoons sea salt, divided

½ teaspoon freshly ground black pepper, divided

1 head cauliflower, broken into florets

1 head Roasted Garlic (page 230)

1 cup Slow Cooker Caramelized Onions (page 228)

2 tablespoons sugar-free prepared horseradish, or fresh grated
   horseradish root

1. In the crock of a slow cooker, combine the short ribs, mushrooms, carrots, onion, garlic, thyme, mustard, vinegar, 2 cups of Slow Cooker Bone Broth, 1 teaspoon of salt, and ¼ teaspoon of pepper. Cover and cook for 10 hours, until the ribs are soft.

2. In a large pot of water, bring the cauliflower to a boil. Boil until it is soft, about 10 minutes.

3. Drain the cauliflower, and put it back in the pot with the remaining ¼ cup broth, the Roasted Garlic, Slow Cooker Caramelized Onions, and the remaining ½ teaspoon salt and ¼ teaspoon pepper. Using a potato masher, mash the cauliflower.

4. Remove the meat from the slow cooker and set it aside on a platter, tented with foil.

5. Working in batches, add everything else in the slow cooker to a blender or food processor, along with the horseradish. Blend until smooth, taking care to allow the steam to escape as you do.

6. Serve the mashed cauliflower and meat topped with the gravy.

PER SERVING Calories: 396; Total Fat: 16g; Saturated Fat: 6g; Cholesterol: 155mg; Carbohydrates: 9g; Fiber: 3g; Protein: 52g

TRI-TIP ROAST CHIMICHURRI WITH DAIKON RADISH FRIES

Serves 8 / Prep time: 20 minutes / Cook time: 90 minutes

WEEK 2

Originally from Argentina, chimichurri is a green sauce for meat. Tri-tip roast is one of the most flavorful cuts of beef you can roast. Season it liberally with salt and pepper before roasting it. While the roast rests, cook your crispy daikon radish fries for a tasty side.

FOR THE ROAST

1 (3- to 4-pound) beef tri-tip roast
Sea salt
Freshly ground black pepper

FOR THE CHIMICHURRI SAUCE

2 cups fresh Italian parsley, leaves only
4 garlic cloves
¼ cup fresh oregano leaves
¼ cup red wine vinegar
¾ cup extra-virgin olive oil
½ teaspoon sea salt
¼ teaspoon freshly ground black pepper

FOR THE DAIKON RADISH FRIES

1 large daikon radish, peeled and cut into ¼-inch-thick julienne
2 tablespoons melted animal fat, such as duck fat or lard
Sea salt

TO MAKE THE ROAST

1. An hour before cooking, put the roast out on the counter and let it come to room temperature.

2. Preheat the oven to 425°F.

3. Season the roast with salt and pepper, and put it on a baking sheet.

4. Put the roast in the oven and lower the temperature to 350°F. Roast for 30 to 45 minutes, until it reaches 135° on an instant-read thermometer.

5. Remove the roast from the oven and set it aside, tented with foil, while you prepare the sauce and the fries.

TO MAKE THE CHIMICHURRI SAUCE

1. In a food processor fitted with a chopping blade, pulse the parsley, garlic, oregano, vinegar, olive oil, salt, and pepper until they are well chopped and combined.

2. Set the sauce aside to let the flavors blend.

TO MAKE THE DAIKON RADISH FRIES

1. For the last half hour the meat is cooking, in a large bowl, soak the radishes in cold water. Remove from the water and pat dry.

2. Turn the oven up to 475°F when you remove the roast.

3. In a large bowl, toss the radishes with the animal fat and salt. Put them on a baking sheet and bake for 30 minutes, turning about halfway through the cooking.

4. Slice the roast against the grain. Top the roast with the chimichurri sauce, and serve with the fries on the side.

Ingredient tip: Slicing the roast against the grain shortens the fibers, making it much more tender than if you slice with the grain of the meat.

PER SERVING Calories: 425; Total Fat: 30g; Saturated Fat: 7g; Cholesterol: 101mg; Carbohydrates: 5g; Fiber: 2g; Protein: 38g

STEAK FAJITAS
WITH ONIONS AND PEPPERS

Serves 8 / Prep time: 20 minutes, plus 8 hours to marinate /
Cook time: 30 minutes

This meat is easy to make ahead and then reheat in the microwave if you're pressed for time on weeknights. Make the guacamole the day of, because it never keeps very well, since avocado oxidizes so easily.

Juice of 3 limes
¼ cup extra-virgin olive oil
1 jalapeño pepper, seeded and minced
3 garlic cloves, minced
5 scallions, sliced
¼ cup fresh cilantro, chopped
1 teaspoon sea salt
¼ teaspoon freshly ground black pepper
1 (3-pound) skirt steak
2 tablespoons coconut oil
1 green bell pepper, sliced
1 red bell pepper, sliced
1 onion, sliced
Butter lettuce leaves
2 cups Guacamole (page 106)

1. In the bowl of a food processor, pulse the lime juice, olive oil, jalapeño, garlic, scallions, cilantro, salt, and pepper for 20 one-second pulses to combine.

2. Using a rubber scraper, scrape all but 2 tablespoons of the mixture into a large resealable storage bag. Put the remaining 2 tablespoons in a small container. Cover it and refrigerate it.

3. Add the skirt steak to the bag. Seal and massage the bag to coat the steak with the marinade.

4. Refrigerate and marinate for 4 to 8 hours in the refrigerator.

5. Remove the steak from the marinade, wiping away any excess marinade with a paper towel.

6. In a large sauté pan over medium-high heat, heat the coconut oil until it shimmers. Add the skirt steak and cook until it is medium-rare, about 7 minutes per side.

7. Remove the steak from the pan, and allow it to rest for 10 minutes. Meanwhile, add the green and red pepper and the onion to the pan and cook, stirring frequently, until they are soft, about 6 minutes.

8. Slice the steak on the diagonal into ½-inch-thick strips. Add them to the pan along with the reserved marinade. Cook, stirring constantly, until the marinade coats the meat and vegetables.

9. Serve with butter lettuce leaves as tortillas and top with Guacamole.

Cooking tip: To slice "on the diagonal" means to cut across at about a 45° angle.

PER SERVING Calories: 553; Total Fat: 37g; Saturated Fat: 13g; Cholesterol: 100mg; Carbohydrates: 8g; Fiber: 5g; Protein: 47g

GREEK-STYLE LAMB BURGERS WITH RED ONION QUICK PICKLE, GARLIC MAYONNAISE, AND CUCUMBER SALAD

Serves 4 / Prep time: 20 minutes / Cook time: 30 minutes

WEEK 1 / WEEK 4

These delicious burgers have Mediterranean seasoning. Instead of using a bun, serve them on a bed of cucumber salad topped with a quick pickle of red onions and some homemade garlic mayonnaise. While the recipe calls for roasting the burgers, you can also grill them.

FOR THE QUICK PICKLE

½ cup red wine vinegar

½ teaspoon sea salt

½ red onion, thinly sliced

FOR THE LAMB BURGERS

1 pound ground lamb

4 garlic cloves, minced

2 teaspoons chopped fresh oregano

1 teaspoon chopped fresh rosemary

½ teaspoon sea salt

¼ teaspoon freshly ground black pepper

FOR THE GARLIC MAYONNAISE

½ cup Homemade Mayonnaise (page 229)

Juice and zest of ½ lemon

1 garlic clove, minced

FOR THE CUCUMBER SALAD

2 medium cucumbers, chopped

2 cups baby arugula

3 tablespoons extra-virgin olive oil

Juice and zest of ½ lemon

1 tablespoon red wine vinegar

1 teaspoon chopped fresh oregano

¼ teaspoon sea salt

¼ teaspoon freshly ground black pepper

TO MAKE THE QUICK PICKLE

1. In a small bowl, whisk together the vinegar and salt. Stir in the red onion.

2. Cover and refrigerate for 30 minutes to 1 hour.

TO MAKE THE LAMB BURGERS

1. Preheat the oven to 400°F.

2. Put a baking rack over a baking sheet.

3. In a large bowl, stir together the ground lamb, garlic, oregano, rosemary, salt, and pepper.

4. Form the mixture into 4 patties, and put them on the rack.

5. Bake until the lamb reaches 165°F, about 30 minutes.

TO MAKE THE GARLIC MAYONNAISE

1. In a small bowl, whisk together the Homemade Mayonnaise, lemon juice, lemon zest, and garlic.

2. Set aside to let the flavors blend.

TO MAKE THE CUCUMBER SALAD

1. In a large bowl, toss together the cucumbers and arugula.

2. In a small bowl, whisk together the olive oil, lemon juice, lemon zest, vinegar, oregano, salt, and pepper.

3. Pour over the salad, and toss to combine. ▸

**GREEK-STYLE LAMB BURGERS WITH RED ONION QUICK PICKLE,
GARLIC MAYONNAISE, AND CUCUMBER SALAD** *continued*

TO ASSEMBLE

1. Spoon the cucumber salad onto four plates.

2. Top each with a lamb burger, 2 tablespoons of the mayonnaise, and some red onions (removed from the vinegar), and serve.

Cooking tip: One of the best ways to finely mince garlic so it mixes easily and evenly into the mayonnaise is to use a garlic press. These handy gadgets are great to own if you plan to mince lots of garlic.

PER SERVING Calories: 460; Total Fat: 29g; Saturated Fat: 6g; Cholesterol: 110mg; Carbohydrates: 17g; Fiber: 2g; Protein: 40g

MUSTARD AND HERB LEG OF LAMB

Serves 12 / Prep time: 5 minutes / Cook time: 80 minutes

The recipe doesn't require much hands-on time. It's just a quick prep of the marinade and then cooking time—when you can be doing other things. The lamb has lots of leftovers, which make for quick lunches and dinners. You can also make it ahead and reheat it. Serve this tasty, easy-to-prepare leg of lamb with Spinach Salad with Warm Bacon Vinaigrette (page 136). You can prepare the salad while the lamb rests.

NIGHTSHADE-FREE

NUT-FREE

MAKE-AHEAD

1 bunch chives
1 cup fresh basil leaves
1 teaspoon sea salt
¼ teaspoon freshly ground black pepper
6 garlic cloves
3 tablespoons Dijon mustard
2 tablespoons extra-virgin olive oil
1 tablespoon red wine vinegar
1 (5-pound) leg of lamb

1. Preheat the oven to 400°F.

2. In the bowl of a food processor, process the chives, basil, salt, pepper, garlic, mustard, olive oil, and vinegar until it forms a paste, about 30 seconds.

3. Rub the mixture all over the leg of lamb, and put it in a large roasting pan.

4. Roast for 20 minutes. Then turn the heat down to 300°F and continue roasting for about 1 hour more, about 12 minutes per pound. Remove from the oven when the roast reaches an internal temperature of 145°F.

5. Allow the lamb to rest, tented with foil, for about 20 minutes before carving and serving.

PER SERVING Calories: 366; Total Fat: 15g; Saturated Fat: 5g; Cholesterol: 164mg; Carbohydrates: 1g; Fiber: 0g; Protein: 54g

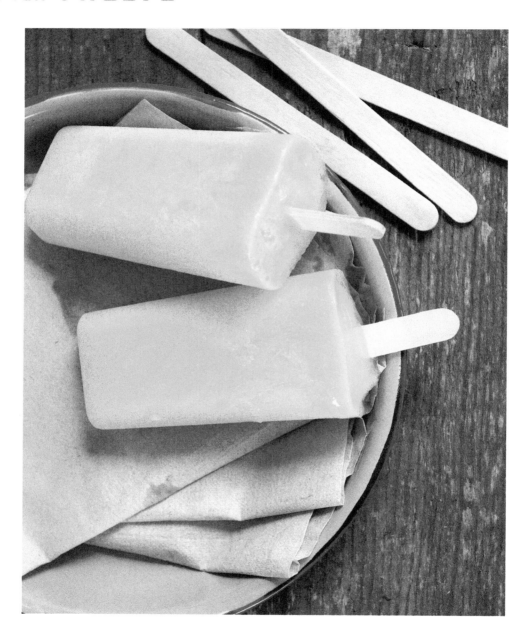

CHAPTER TWELVE

DESSERTS

FRUIT KEBABS
WITH YOGURT DIPPING SAUCE

Serves 8 / Prep time: 10 minutes

NIGHTSHADE-
FREE

NUT-FREE

VEGAN

MAKE-AHEAD

QUICK &
EASY

These fruit kebabs are simple, light, and a lot of fun. You can use any seasonal fruits you wish for the kebabs, so don't feel limited to those listed here. Be sure you select an unsweetened plain coconut yogurt (also called cultured coconut milk) for the dipping sauce.

2 cups pineapple chunks

2 cups large strawberries, halved

2 bananas, sliced

1 cup plain unsweetened coconut yogurt

½ teaspoon stevia

½ teaspoon ground cinnamon

¼ teaspoon ground nutmeg

Pinch of salt

1. Thread the pineapples, strawberries, and bananas in an alternating pattern onto wooden skewers.

2. In a small bowl, whisk together the yogurt, stevia, cinnamon, nutmeg, and salt.

3. Serve the skewers on a platter with the dipping sauce.

PER SERVING Calories: 72; Total Fat: 1g; Saturated Fat: 1g; Cholesterol: 0mg; Carbohydrates: 17g; Fiber: 3g; Protein: 1g

FROZEN PEACHES AND CREAM BARS

Serves 6 / Prep time: 5 minutes, plus 8 hours to freeze

You can use either fresh or frozen peaches in this recipe, although fresh seasonal peaches add a lot more flavor to the dessert. If you don't have ice pop molds, you can use paper cups. Once you pour the mixture into the cups, cover them with a piece of foil and push the stick through the foil into the cup.

8 ounces plain unsweetened coconut yogurt

6 peaches, pitted and chopped

1 cup coconut milk

½ teaspoon stevia

1. In a blender or food processor, blend the yogurt, peaches, coconut milk, and stevia until smooth, about 60 seconds.

2. Pour the mixture into ice pop molds and insert popsicle sticks. Freeze for 8 hours, and serve.

PER SERVING Calories: 172; Total Fat: 11g; Saturated Fat: 10g; Cholesterol: 0mg; Carbohydrates: 17g; Fiber: 2g; Protein: 3g

NIGHTSHADE-FREE

NUT-FREE

VEGAN

QUICK & EASY

REFRESHING LEMON BLACKBERRY ICE

Serves 4 / Prep time: 10 minutes, plus 8 hours to freeze

Lemons and blackberries make a sweet-tart combination that tastes delicious, especially as an ice. You can make the ice a week ahead of time, and then break it up and blend it just before serving.

NIGHTSHADE-FREE

NUT-FREE

VEGAN

QUICK & EASY

1 cup freshly squeezed lemon juice
3 cups blackberries
1 teaspoon stevia

1. In a blender or food processor, blend the lemon juice, blackberries, and stevia until the berries are crushed, about 20 seconds.

2. Pour the mixture into a 9-by-9-inch glass dish lined with parchment paper, and freeze for 8 hours.

3. Break the frozen mixture into pieces, process in a blender or food processor until it has a slushy texture, about 1 minute, and serve.

Substitution tip: For an interesting herbal twist, add ½ teaspoon of chopped fresh thyme to the lemons and blueberries.

PER SERVING Calories: 61; Total Fat: 1g; Saturated Fat: 0g; Cholesterol: 0mg; Carbohydrates: 12g; Fiber: 6g; Protein: 2g

COOL MINT AND HONEYDEW SLUSHY

Serves 2 / Prep time: 10 minutes

Choose honeydew melons at the height of their season in early summer for the best flavor. Melons in season are so sweet, they don't need anything other than their natural flavor for sweetness. Fresh mint leaves add a refreshing twist to this delicious slushy.

1 honeydew melon, rind and seeds removed, cut into chunks

1 cup sparkling water

3 mint leaves, minced

2 cups crushed ice

In a food processor or blender, blend the melon, water, mint, and ice until combined, about 1 minute, and serve.

PER SERVING Calories: 115; Total Fat: 1g; Saturated Fat: 0g; Cholesterol: 0mg; Carbohydrates: 30g; Fiber: 3g; Protein: 1g

FODMAP-
FREE

NIGHTSHADE-
FREE

NUT-FREE

VEGAN

QUICK &
EASY

COCONUT CREAM WITH SUMMER BERRIES

Serves 2 / Prep time: 10 minutes

This recipe keeps it light and fresh. It also requires no cooking and is very versatile. You can substitute any berries you wish, for a tasty treat. The coconut milk contains fat, so even though the dessert is light, it is also very satisfying.

½ cup Coconut Cream (page 235)

¼ teaspoon stevia

1 cup strawberries, sliced

1 cup blueberries

1 cup raspberries

1. In a small bowl, whisk the coconut cream and stevia until well combined.

2. In a medium bowl, mix the strawberries, blueberries, and raspberries.

3. Spoon the berries into two bowls, top them with the Coconut Cream, and serve.

PER SERVING Calories: 357; Total Fat: 28g; Saturated Fat: 24g; Cholesterol: 0mg; Carbohydrates: 30g; Fiber: 10g; Protein: 4g

FODMAP-FREE

NIGHTSHADE-FREE

NUT-FREE

VEGAN

QUICK & EASY

CHOCOLATE-COVERED BLUEBERRY-COCONUT BARS

Serves 6 / Prep time: 5 minutes, plus 8 hours to freeze /
Cook time: 10 minutes

Use wild organic frozen blueberries in this recipe. These small blueberries are really flavorful. You can also use fresh blueberries if you wish. Coconut oil solidifies at room temperature, giving the chocolate coating the nice bite you love in ice cream bars.

2 cups frozen organic wild blueberries

2 cups coconut milk

8 ounces plain unsweetened coconut milk yogurt

1½ teaspoons stevia, divided

2 ounces unsweetened chocolate

½ cup coconut oil

1 cup shredded coconut, unsweetened

NIGHTSHADE-FREE

NUT-FREE

VEGAN

MAKE-AHEAD

QUICK & EASY

1. In a blender or food processor, blend the blueberries, coconut milk, yogurt, and ¾ teaspoon of stevia until well mixed, about 60 seconds.

2. Pour the mixture into ice pop molds (or paper cups), insert the sticks, and freeze for 8 hours.

3. Line a plate with parchment paper.

4. In a small pan over low heat, melt the chocolate and coconut oil. Stir in the remaining ¾ teaspoon stevia. Remove from the heat and allow to cool slightly.

5. Spread the shredded coconut on a plate in a thin layer.

6. Unmold the frozen pops, and dip them in the chocolate. Roll them in the coconut, and lay them on the parchment paper.

7. Freeze until the chocolate hardens completely and serve.

PER SERVING Calories: 480; Total Fat: 48g; Saturated Fat: 41g; Cholesterol: 0mg; Carbohydrates: 18g; Fiber: 7g; Protein: 4g

CHOCOLATE BROWNIE BITES

Makes 8 bites / Prep time: 5 minutes

These no-bake brownie bites are full of chocolaty goodness. They get their sweetness from dates, which add a nice sticky, gooey character. You can substitute walnuts or hazelnuts for the pecans if you wish.

NIGHTSHADE-
FREE

VEGAN

MAKE-AHEAD

QUICK &
EASY

1½ cups pecans
1 cup dates, pitted
Pinch of salt
½ teaspoon vanilla extract
Zest of ½ orange
⅓ cup unsweetened cocoa powder

1. In the bowl of a food processor fitted with a chopping blade, pulse the pecans for 20 one-second pulses, until they form a meal.

2. Add the dates, salt, vanilla, orange zest, and cocoa powder, and process until well combined, 1 to 2 minutes.

3. Roll the mixture into small balls, and refrigerate until you're ready to serve.

PER SERVING Calories: 196; Total Fat: 14g; Saturated Fat: 1g; Cholesterol: 0mg; Carbohydrates: 21g; Fiber: 5g; Protein: 3g

CHOCOLATE-DIPPED STRAWBERRIES

Makes 12 berries / Prep time: 5 minutes, plus more to refrigerate /
Cook time: 5 minutes

During strawberry season in June, you can find delicious berries. Look for deep red strawberries with a lovely uniform shape. Leave the stems in place to give these chocolate-dipped strawberries a classic look.

½ cup coconut oil

2 ounces unsweetened chocolate

1 teaspoon stevia

12 large strawberries

1. Line a plate or tray with parchment paper.

2. In a small saucepan over low heat, melt the coconut oil, chocolate, and stevia, stirring constantly.

3. Holding the strawberries at the stem end, dip them ¾ of the way into the chocolate. Allow the extra chocolate to drip away from the end of the berries.

4. Put the berries on the prepared plate, refrigerate them to harden the chocolate, and serve.

Substitution tip: Use orange segments or apples in place of the strawberries.

PER SERVING (1 BERRY) Calories: 106; Total Fat: 12g; Saturated Fat: 9g; Cholesterol: 0mg; Carbohydrates: 2g; Fiber: 1g; Protein: 1g

NIGHTSHADE-FREE

NUT-FREE

VEGAN

MAKE-AHEAD

QUICK & EASY

AVOCADO-CHOCOLATE-ORANGE MOUSSE

Serves 4 / Prep time: 5 minutes, plus more to chill

The secret to this smooth, creamy mousse is avocado. Not only does it give the mousse a wonderful texture, but it also adds fiber and vitamins. You can make this mousse ahead of time and chill it. Serve within 24 hours for best results.

2 ripe avocados, halved, peeled, and pitted
⅓ cup unsweetened cocoa powder
⅓ cup coconut milk
Juice and zest of ½ orange
1 teaspoon stevia
½ teaspoon ground cinnamon
Dash sea salt

1. In the bowl of a food processor, process the avocados, cocoa powder, coconut milk, orange juice, orange zest, stevia, cinnamon, and salt until smooth, about 1 minute.
2. Chill before serving.

Ingredient tip: Select soft avocados that aren't overripe. The perfect avocado will yield to mild pressure with the thumb. Pop off the stem on the end, and look at the fruit underneath. If it is green and the avocado is soft, then it's just right.

PER SERVING Calories: 268; Total Fat: 25g; Saturated Fat: 9g; Cholesterol: 0mg; Carbohydrates: 14g; Fiber: 10g; Protein: 4g

NIGHTSHADE-FREE

NUT-FREE

VEGAN

MAKE-AHEAD

QUICK & EASY

ORANGE POACHED PEARS
WITH NUTMEG

Serves 2 / Prep time: 10 minutes / Cook time: 30 minutes

With orange and spices, this is a delicious fall dessert when pears are in season. While you can choose any pears you wish, a slightly under-ripe Bosc pear is especially good in this tasty dessert. The juice will turn into syrup while it simmers, so you can use it as a sauce.

1½ cups orange juice

¼ teaspoon stevia

¼ teaspoon fresh grated nutmeg

2 pears, halved, peeled, and cored

○ NIGHTSHADE-FREE

○ NUT-FREE

○ VEGAN

1. In a small saucepan over medium heat, bring the orange juice, stevia, and nutmeg to a simmer.

2. Add the pears to the juice. Turn frequently, allowing them to simmer, until they are soft, about 30 minutes.

3. Serve in a bowl with the juice spooned over the top.

Ingredient tip: Fresh nutmeg has a delicious flavor that is different from ground nutmeg. In the spice aisle, look for whole nutmeg seeds. The best tool for grating them is a rasp-style grater.

PER SERVING Calories: 206; Total Fat: 1g; Saturated Fat: 0g; Cholesterol: 0mg; Carbohydrates: 51g; Fiber: 7g; Protein: 2g

VANILLA-CHAMOMILE POACHED PLUMS

Serves 4 / Prep time: 10 minutes / Cook time: 10 minutes

Use a vanilla bean to add a true vanilla flavor to these poached plums. You can also use juicy pluots, a hybrid of plums and apricots, in this recipe. Pluots are sweeter than plums but still have a nice tangy flavor.

2 cups brewed chamomile tea
½ teaspoon stevia
Seeds of 1 vanilla bean
8 plums, halved and pitted

1. In a small saucepan over medium heat, bring the tea, stevia, and vanilla to a simmer.

2. Add the plums and cook, turning frequently, until they are soft, 10 to 15 minutes.

3. Serve warm.

Cooking tip: To get the vanilla beans out of the pod, halve the pod lengthwise. Then, using the tip of your knife, scrape the beans from the pod directly into the saucepan.

PER SERVING Calories: 40; Total Fat: 0g; Saturated Fat: 0g; Cholesterol: 0mg; Carbohydrates: 10g; Fiber: 1g; Protein: 1g

NIGHTSHADE-FREE

NUT-FREE

VEGAN

QUICK & EASY

APPLE-PEAR SAUCE

Serves 4 / Prep time: 20 minutes / Cook time: 20 minutes

Use a sweet-tart apple such as a Granny Smith or Honeycrisp for this sauce. For pears, choose an Anjou or Bosc pear. Peel the apples and pears. While this recipe doesn't call for any sweetener, you can adjust the sweetness by adding a little stevia.

3 apples, peeled, cored, and sliced

3 pears, peeled, cored, and sliced

¼ cup water

Juice of ½ lemon

¼ teaspoon ground ginger

1 teaspoon ground cinnamon

¼ teaspoon ground nutmeg

NIGHTSHADE-FREE

NUT-FREE

VEGAN

MAKE-AHEAD

1. In a small saucepan over medium heat, bring the apples, pears, water, lemon juice, ginger, cinnamon, and nutmeg to a simmer.

2. Cook, stirring frequently, until the apples and pears are soft, about 20 minutes.

3. Serve spooned over Pumpkin Waffles (page 82) or a dessert.

PER SERVING Calories: 164; Total Fat: 1g; Saturated Fat: 0g; Cholesterol: 0mg; Carbohydrates: 43g; Fiber: 9g; Protein: 1g

CRANBERRY-ORANGE COMPOTE

Serves 4 / Prep time: 5 minutes / Cook time: 20 minutes

Who says cranberries are just for the holidays? When combined with orange and spices, this compote makes a delicious end to a meal. Of course, you may love this recipe so much it also becomes your go-to holiday cranberry sauce.

NIGHTSHADE-FREE

NUT-FREE

VEGAN

MAKE-AHEAD

QUICK & EASY

16 ounces fresh cranberries

Juice and zest of 1 orange

½ teaspoon stevia

½ teaspoon ground cinnamon

½ teaspoon fresh grated ginger

Pinch sea salt

1. In a large pot over medium-high heat, heat the cranberries, orange juice, orange zest, stevia, cinnamon, ginger, and salt, stirring frequently, until the cranberries pop and and the sauce thickens, about 20 minutes.

2. Cool before serving.

PER SERVING Calories: 77; Total Fat: 0g; Saturated Fat: 0g; Cholesterol: 0mg; Carbohydrates: 14g; Fiber: 4g; Protein: 7g

ORANGE-SCENTED MERINGUE COOKIES

Makes 12 cookies / Prep time: 20 minutes / Cook time: 60 minutes

These cookies keep well, as long as you store them in an airtight container at room temperature. The cooking time and temperature are slow and low to get the cookies to the right crisp consistency. If you don't like orange, you can leave it out and just use vanilla bean seeds or cinnamon instead.

3 egg whites
¼ teaspoon cream of tartar
½ teaspoon stevia
Zest of ½ orange

FODMAP-FREE

NIGHTSHADE-FREE

NUT-FREE

VEGETARIAN

MAKE-AHEAD

1. Preheat the oven to 215°F.

2. Line a baking sheet with parchment paper.

3. In a large bowl, beat the egg whites until they begin to stiffen, about 5 minutes.

4. Add the cream of tartar, stevia, and orange zest, and continue beating until stiff peaks form, another 5 minutes.

5. Drop the cookies by the spoonful onto the prepared baking sheet. Bake the cookies until they are browned and crisped, 50 minutes to 1 hour.

6. Remove the cookies from the baking sheet with a spatula, and cool them on a wire rack before serving.

Ingredient tip: To get the egg whites to stiff peaks, it is best to start with them at room temperature. Be sure you don't get any fat in the egg whites, or they will not beat to stiff peaks.

PER SERVING (1 COOKIE) Calories: 10; Total Fat: 0g; Saturated Fat: 0g; Cholesterol: 0mg; Carbohydrates: 0g; Fiber: 0g; Protein: 1g

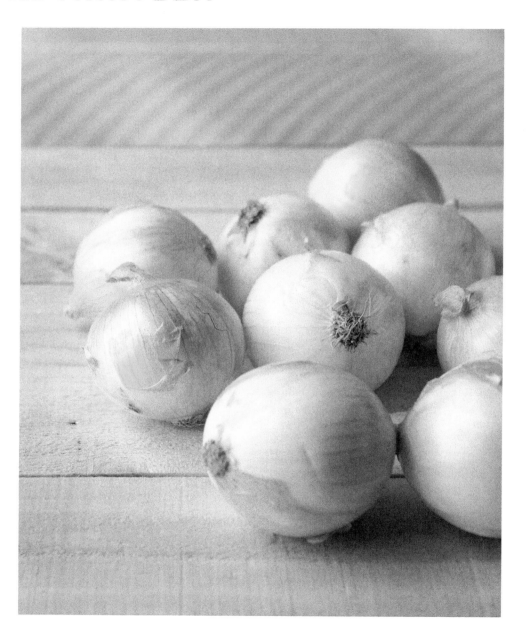

KITCHEN STAPLES

SLOW COOKER BONE BROTH

Makes 2 quarts / Prep time: 10 minutes / Cook time: 12 to 24 hours

NIGHTSHADE-
FREE

NUT-FREE

MAKE-AHEAD

You can use this recipe for any type of broth, such as chicken, beef, or duck. Use bones with just a little meat left on them, or with no meat at all. You can use cooked bones, such as a roasted turkey carcass, or raw bones, such as beef marrow bones. In my house, I don't throw any bones away, saving them to make broth. Adjust the amounts and types of seasonings, aromatic vegetables, and herbs to meet your needs. The broth will keep in the refrigerator for three to five days or in the freezer for up to a year. I make broth once or twice a week and keep a large supply in my freezer.

3 to 5 pounds animal bones

1 sprig rosemary

10 peppercorns

1 onion, unpeeled, quartered

2 carrots, unpeeled, chopped

1 celery stalk, chopped

1 teaspoon sea salt

4 garlic cloves, smashed

2 to 3 quarts water, or enough to cover the bones and vegetables

1. In the crock of a large slow cooker, combine the bones, rosemary, peppercorns, onion, carrots, celery, salt, garlic, and water. Cover and cook on high for 12 to 24 hours. Poultry is usually finished after 12 hours, while beef bones may need closer to 24 hours.

2. Using a sieve, strain the broth into a large container to remove and discard the solids. Cover the container, and refrigerate it overnight.

3. In the morning, skim the congealed fat from the top of the broth. You can save this rendered fat if you wish for cooking; just keep it refrigerated.

4. Pour the broth into freezer-safe containers that seal tightly. Freeze the broth to use in recipes.

PER SERVING (1 CUP) Calories: 38; Total Fat: 1g; Saturated Fat: 0g; Cholesterol: 0mg; Carbohydrates: 1g; Fiber: 0g; Protein: 5g

SLOW COOKER VEGETABLE BROTH

Makes 2 to 3 quarts / Prep time: 10 minutes / Cook time: 12 to 24 hours

Making vegetable broth doesn't take a lot of time, and it's a great way to use up vegetable trimmings you would normally discard. I keep a large resealable storage bag of vegetable trimmings in my freezer that I pull out and use whenever I want to make broth. Save trimmings from onions, carrot peels, celery tops, leek tops, garlic trimmings, and mushroom stems. Avoid vegetables like bell peppers, which may give a bitter flavor to the broth. Add aromatic herbs such as thyme, parsley, or rosemary, along with salt, peppercorns, and enough water to cover the vegetable trimmings. You can also make this simple broth with whole vegetables. To save time, just chop the vegetables very roughly.

NIGHTSHADE-FREE

NUT-FREE

VEGAN

MAKE-AHEAD

3 onions, peels on, quartered

6 garlic cloves, smashed

3 carrots, roughly chopped

3 celery stalks, including leaves, roughly chopped

8 ounces mushrooms

3 sprigs fresh thyme

2 sprigs fresh parsley

1 teaspoon sea salt

10 peppercorns

2 to 3 quarts water, or enough to cover the vegetables

1. In the crock of a large slow cooker, combine the onions, garlic, carrots, celery, mushrooms, thyme, parsley, salt, peppercorns, and water. Cover and cook on low for 12 hours.

2. Using a sieve, strain the broth into a large container to remove and discard the solids.

3. Pour the broth into freezer-safe containers that seal tightly. Freeze the broth to use in recipes.

PER SERVING (1 CUP) Calories: 38; Total Fat: 0g; Saturated Fat: 0g; Cholesterol: 0mg; Carbohydrates: 1g; Fiber: 0g; Protein: 5g

SLOW COOKER CARAMELIZED ONIONS

Makes 2 cups / Prep time: 10 minutes / Cook time: 15 hours

Caramelized onions can add deep savory, sweet, and umami flavors to dishes. Making them on the stove top takes about 45 minutes for a batch. You can also make a large batch in a slow cooker and freeze them so you have them to use whenever you'd like.

5 onions, peeled and sliced

3 tablespoons melted animal fat

½ teaspoon sea salt

NIGHTSHADE-
FREE

NUT-FREE

MAKE-AHEAD

1. In the crock of a large slow cooker, toss the onions, animal fat, and salt.

2. Cover the slow cooker, and turn it on low for 10 hours.

3. Remove the lid from the slow cooker, and continue cooking for another 3 to 5 hours to allow the liquid to evaporate.

4. Store the onions in airtight containers in the refrigerator or freezer.

Time-saving tip: If you don't want to cook the onions for the extra 3 to 5 hours to evaporate the liquid, you could strain them through a sieve instead.

PER SERVING (¼ CUP) Calories: 71; Total Fat: 5g; Saturated Fat: 2g; Cholesterol: 5mg; Carbohydrates: 7g; Fiber: 2g; Protein: 1g

HOMEMADE MAYONNAISE

Makes 1½ cups / Prep time: 10 minutes

Commercial mayonnaise often uses industrial seed oils. Many commercial mayonnaises also contain sugar, often in the form of high-fructose corn syrup. Making your own mayonnaise is quick and easy, particularly if you have a food processor, blender, or immersion blender. Even if you don't have any of this equipment, you can still make mayonnaise using a whisk; it just takes longer.

2 egg yolks

½ teaspoon sea salt

1 tablespoon apple cider vinegar

¾ cup avocado oil

¾ cup extra-virgin olive oil

1. In the bowl of a food processor fitted with a chopping blade or a blender, begin processing the egg yolks, salt, and apple cider vinegar.

2. Through the chute of the processor, add the avocado oil and olive oil, a drop at a time, until you've incorporated 20 drops. Then continue adding the oil in a thin stream while the food processor or blender runs. Continue until all the oil is incorporated.

3. The mayonnaise will keep in the refrigerator for up to 1 week.

PER SERVING (1 TABLESPOON) Calories: 57; Total Fat: 5g; Saturated Fat: 1g; Cholesterol: 0mg; Carbohydrates: 2g; Fiber: 0g; Protein: 0g

FODMAP-FREE

NIGHTSHADE-FREE

NUT-FREE

VEGETARIAN

MAKE-AHEAD

QUICK & EASY

ROASTED GARLIC

Makes 4 heads of garlic / Prep time: 5 minutes / Cook time: 60 minutes

Use roasted garlic to add a deep, rich, caramelized flavor to soups, stews, and sauces. To remove the roasted garlic cloves from the head, squeeze the head over a small dish. Roast the garlic in bulk, and freeze the squeezed cloves until you'd like to use them.

NIGHTSHADE-FREE

NUT-FREE

VEGAN

MAKE-AHEAD

4 garlic heads, tops cut off to expose the cloves
2 tablespoons melted animal fat
¼ teaspoon sea salt

1. Preheat the oven to 350°F.
2. In a glass bread pan, place the garlic cloves cut-side up. Drizzle the cloves with the fat, and sprinkle them with the salt.
3. Cover with foil and roast until soft, about 60 minutes.
4. Squeeze the garlic cloves into an airtight container and refrigerate for up to a week or freeze for up to a year.

PER SERVING (1 HEAD) Calories: 75; Total Fat: 7g; Saturated Fat: 3g; Cholesterol: 6mg; Carbohydrates: 3g; Fiber 0g; Protein: 0g

CAULIFLOWER "RICE"

Makes 6 cups / Prep time: 10 minutes / Cook time: 5 minutes

Cauliflower "rice" is a common replacement for white or brown rice. It's easy to prepare, and you can freeze it in one-cup portions in a zipper bag in the freezer. If you don't have a food processor, you can use a large chef's knife to finely chop the cauliflower florets to a ricelike consistency. You can also grate the cauliflower on a cheese grater.

FOR THE RICE

1 head cauliflower, broken into florets

FOR COOKING 1 CUP OF THE RICE

2 tablespoons coconut oil

¼ teaspoon sea salt

TO MAKE THE RICE

In the bowl of a food processor fitted with a chopping blade, pulse the cauliflower for 20 to 30 one-second pulses, until the cauliflower is chopped into a ricelike texture.

TO COOK 1 CUP OF THE RICE

In a large sauté pan over medium-high heat, heat the coconut oil until it shimmers. Add 1 cup of the cauliflower and cook, stirring frequently, until it is soft, about 5 minutes. Repeat with the remaining cauliflower.

Time-saving tip: Chop up the cauliflower ahead and freeze it uncooked in 1-cup-size portions. Then cook it before using it in a recipe.

PER SERVING (1 CUP) Calories: 265; Total Fat: 27g; Saturated Fat: 4g; Cholesterol: 0mg; Carbohydrates: 5g; Fiber: 3g; Protein: 2g

NIGHTSHADE-FREE

NUT-FREE

VEGAN

MAKE-AHEAD

QUICK & EASY

ZUCCHINI "SPAGHETTI"

Serves 4 / Prep time: 10 minutes / Cook time: 5 minutes

Replace pasta in recipes with this zucchini "spaghetti." The great thing about it is that you can cut the zucchini into spaghetti strips or leave it as ribbons for a different shape. Leave the peel on the zucchini for additional color.

FODMAP-
FREE

NIGHTSHADE-
FREE

NUT-FREE

VEGAN

QUICK &
EASY

6 medium zucchini

2 tablespoons coconut oil

¼ teaspoon sea salt

¼ cup water

1. Using a vegetable peeler, cut the zucchini into long ribbons.

2. Using a paring knife, cut the ribbons lengthwise into thin strips.

3. In a large sauté pan over medium-high heat, heat the coconut oil until it shimmers.

4. Add the zucchini and cook, stirring constantly, for 3 minutes.

5. Add the salt and water and continue to cook, stirring occasionally, until the zucchini softens, about 5 minutes more. Drain before serving.

Time-saving tip: To save time, put the zucchini in ¼ cup of water with ¼ teaspoon of salt in a covered, microwave-safe dish. Microwave for 2 minutes, and drain before serving.

PER SERVING (1 CUP) Calories: 106; Total Fat: 7g; Saturated Fat: 6g; Cholesterol: 0mg; Carbohydrates: 10g; Fiber: 3g; Protein: 2g

HARDBOILED EGGS

Makes 8 eggs / Cook time: 14 minutes

Hardboiled eggs are a wonderful and affordable source of protein. Have them as a snack, or use them in recipes and salads. Eggs that are slightly older peel much more easily than very fresh eggs, so try to use eggs that are at least a week old.

8 eggs
Pinch sea salt

1. In a large saucepan, put the eggs in a single layer and add water to cover them by 1 inch.

2. Cover the pan, and put it on the stove. Turn the heat to medium-high and bring the eggs to a boil.

3. Remove the pan from the heat. Allow them to sit, covered, in the hot water for 14 minutes.

4. Remove the eggs from the water, and plunge them into a bowl of ice water to stop them cooking. The eggs will keep in the refrigerator, unpeeled, for 1 to 2 weeks.

PER SERVING (1 EGG) Calories: 63; Total Fat: 4g; Saturated Fat: 1g; Cholesterol: 163mg; Carbohydrates: 0g; Fiber: 0g; Protein: 6g

FODMAP-FREE

NIGHTSHADE-FREE

NUT-FREE

VEGETARIAN

MAKE-AHEAD

QUICK & EASY

ITALIAN SAUSAGE

Makes 2 cups / Prep time: 10 minutes

Most commercial Italian sausages contain sugar. This recipe provides a great way to have all the flavor of bulk Italian sausage without the sugar. If you aren't sensitive to nightshades and you really like spicier Italian sausage, add up to ½ teaspoon of crushed red pepper flakes.

NIGHTSHADE-FREE

NUT-FREE

MAKE-AHEAD

QUICK & EASY

1 pound ground pork
2 tablespoons red wine vinegar
2 teaspoons garlic powder
2 teaspoons onion powder
2 teaspoons dried basil
2 teaspoons dried parsley
1 teaspoon crushed fennel seeds
⅛ teaspoon dried oregano
1 teaspoon sea salt
½ teaspoon freshly ground black pepper

1. In a large bowl, mix together the pork, vinegar, garlic powder, onion powder, basil, parsley, fennel seeds, oregano, salt, and pepper until well mixed.

2. Store any uncooked sausage in a tightly sealed container in the refrigerator for up to 3 days (or up until the noted expiration date of the ground pork, if earlier).

Cooking tip: Use this sausage in one of the delicious recipes that call for it throughout the book, or form patties and fry them up at breakfast.

PER SERVING Calories: 174; Total Fat: 4g; Saturated Fat: 2g; Cholesterol: 83mg; Carbohydrates: 2g; Fiber: 0g; Protein: 30g

COCONUT CREAM

Makes ¼ to ½ cup / Prep time: 5 minutes

Coconut cream is a great substitute for whipped cream, and it is so easy to make. All you need is a can of full-fat coconut milk (don't use light coconut milk), a refrigerator, a spoon, and a can opener. Then you can use this delicious cream to top berries or in other recipes.

1 (14-ounce) can full-fat coconut milk

1. Refrigerate the can of coconut milk overnight.
2. In the morning, remove the lid and scoop out the thick cream that has formed on the top, leaving the liquid in the bottom of the can. This top part is the cream.

Ingredient tip: For a sweeter cream, whisk in a pinch of stevia and ¼ teaspoon of vanilla extract.

PER SERVING (¼ CUP) Calories: 138; Total Fat: 14g; Saturated Fat: 13g; Cholesterol: 0mg; Carbohydrates: 3g; Fiber: 1g; Protein: 1g

FODMAP-FREE

NIGHTSHADE-FREE

NUT-FREE

VEGAN

MAKE-AHEAD

QUICK & EASY

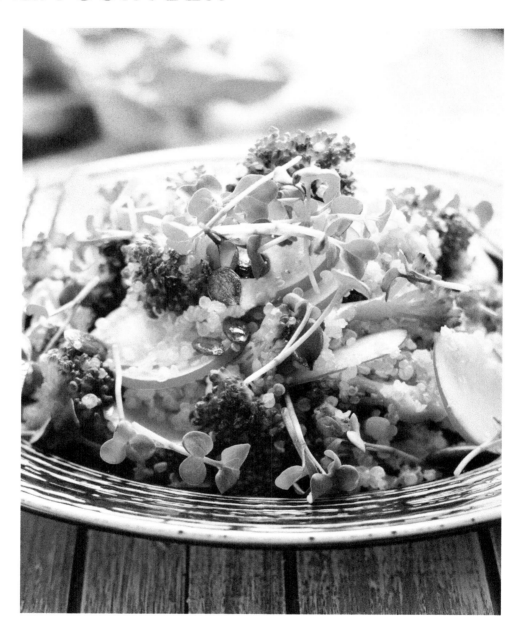

REINTRODUCTION RECIPES

CORN and PEPPER SALAD

Serves 2 / Prep time: 10 minutes

REINTRODUCING CORN

When it's time to reintroduce corn into your diet, this tasty salad is a great way to do it. You can make it ahead and seal it in an airtight container so it's ready to go for lunch the next day. It also makes a delicious side dish.

NUT-FREE

VEGAN

MAKE-AHEAD

QUICK &
EASY

1 (10-ounce) package frozen organic corn, cooked according to package
  directions and cooled

1 red bell pepper, seeded and chopped

½ red onion, finely chopped

2 tablespoons chopped fresh cilantro

¼ cup extra-virgin olive oil

Juice of 2 limes

1 tablespoon apple cider vinegar

¼ teaspoon salt

1 garlic clove, minced

¼ teaspoon ground cumin

1. In a large bowl, stir together the corn, bell pepper, onion, and cilantro.

2. In a small bowl, whisk together the olive oil, lime juice, vinegar, salt, garlic, and cumin.

3. Toss the salad with the dressing and serve.

PER SERVING Calories: 185; Total Fat: 13g; Saturated Fat: 2g; Cholesterol: 0mg; Carbohydrates: 18g; Fiber: 3g; Protein: 2g

SHRIMP TACOS with CORN TORTILLAS

Serves 4 / Prep time: 10 minutes / Cook time: 15 minutes

REINTRODUCING CORN

Shrimp has a lightly sweet flavor that goes very well with the sweetness of corn tortillas. Marinate the shrimp for about thirty minutes before cooking it. Select shrimp that is around 26 to 30 count per pound, which is a medium-size shrimp.

Juice of 2 limes

¼ cup extra-virgin olive oil

¼ teaspoon ground cumin

3 scallions, finely chopped

2 garlic cloves, minced

1 pound shrimp, peeled, deveined, and tails removed

8 soft corn tortillas

2 tablespoons coconut oil

2 cups shredded lettuce

1 avocado, sliced

NIGHTSHADE-FREE

NUT-FREE

QUICK & EASY

1. In a small bowl, whisk together the lime juice, olive oil, cumin, scallions, and garlic. Pour the marinade over the shrimp.

2. While the shrimp marinates, preheat the oven to 350°F.

3. Wrap the corn tortillas in foil, and put them in the preheated oven to warm, about 15 minutes.

4. In a large sauté pan over medium-high heat, heat the coconut oil until it shimmers. Remove the shrimp from the marinade, and add it to the pan. Cook, stirring occasionally, until the shrimp is pink, 5 to 7 minutes.

5. Serve the shrimp with the warm tortillas, shredded lettuce, and avocado slices.

Time-saving tip: Wrap the tortillas in a damp paper towel and microwave them in 30-second increments until they are warm, about 2 minutes.

PER SERVING Calories: 539; Total Fat: 32g; Saturated Fat: 10g; Cholesterol: 239mg; Carbohydrates: 32g; Fiber: 4g; Protein: 30g

CORNMEAL-CRUSTED TILAPIA WITH MANGO SALSA

Serves 4 / Prep time: 10 minutes / Cook time: 15 minutes

REINTRODUCING CORN

NIGHTSHADE-FREE

NUT-FREE

QUICK & EASY

Crusting tilapia in cornmeal gives it a nice crunchy exterior. The corn adds sweetness that pairs well with the fish. The mango salsa avoids nightshades, with no tomatoes or peppers, but it still adds a tasty Latin flair to this dish. If you'd like a little heat and you aren't sensitive to nightshades, add one diced jalapeño pepper.

½ cup cornmeal
½ teaspoon sea salt
¼ teaspoon freshly ground black pepper
4 (4-ounce) tilapia fillets
2 tablespoons coconut oil
2 mangoes, peeled, pitted, and cubed
½ red onion, finely chopped
2 tablespoons chopped fresh cilantro
Juice of 1 lime

1. In a small bowl, toss together the cornmeal, salt, and pepper.
2. Coat the fish fillets in the cornmeal crust.
3. In a large sauté pan over medium-high heat, heat the coconut oil until it shimmers. Add the fish and cook until it is crisp and cooked through, about 4 minutes per side.
4. In a small bowl, mix together the mangoes, red onion, cilantro, and lime juice. Spoon the salsa onto each plate, lay a piece of fish on top of it, and serve.

PER SERVING Calories: 339; Total Fat: 11g; Saturated Fat: 7g; Cholesterol: 67mg; Carbohydrates: 31g; Fiber: 3g; Protein: 31g

BACON, LETTUCE, TOMATO, AND AVOCADO SANDWICH

Serves 1 / Prep time: 10 minutes / Cook time: 10 minutes

REINTRODUCING GLUTEN

Avocados replace mayonnaise on this classic sandwich. The avocado adds a rich fattiness, and it is also high in vitamins and fiber. Use a seasonal tomato, such as an heirloom tomato, for this sandwich. An in-season tomato makes the flavor so much better. If you haven't yet confirmed that you can tolerate nightshades, just leave off the tomato. Use cucumber instead if you'd like to keep that juicy crunch.

NUT-FREE

QUICK & EASY

2 slices thick-cut bacon

2 slices whole-wheat bread, toasted

¼ avocado, lightly mashed

3 thin slices tomato

2 leaves butter lettuce

1. In a sauté pan over medium-high heat, cook the bacon until it is crisp, 5 to 7 minutes.

2. Spread the avocado on one piece of the toast. Put the bacon on top of the avocado, the tomatoes on top of the bacon, and the lettuce on top of the tomato. Finish with the second piece of toast.

PER SERVING Calories: 370; Total Fat: 22g; Saturated Fat: 6g; Cholesterol: 20mg; Carbohydrates: 30g; Fiber: 8g; Protein: 17g

GYROS WITH PITA BREAD

Serves 8 / Prep time: 15 minutes / Cook time: 60 minutes /
Total time: 1 hour, 45 minutes

REINTRODUCING GLUTEN

NIGHTSHADE-
FREE

NUT-FREE

MAKE-AHEAD

Because this recipe makes so many servings, it's great for a large gathering or to have for dinner, with leftovers for lunch or dinner the next day. Cooking the meat in a water bath makes it less likely to burn and gives it the perfect gyro texture.

1 onion, chopped

8 garlic cloves, divided

2 tablespoons chopped fresh rosemary

1 tablespoon fresh oregano

2 pounds ground lamb

1 teaspoon sea salt

½ teaspoon freshly ground black pepper

1 cup Homemade Mayonnaise (page 229)

8 whole-wheat pitas

4 cups arugula

½ red onion, minced

1. Preheat the oven to 325°F.
2. Fill a 9-by-13-inch glass pan one-third full with hot water, and put it in the oven.
3. In the bowl of a food processor, process the onion for 30 seconds. Scrape the onion onto a tea towel. Twist the tea towel around the onion, and wring out the moisture over the sink so the onion is dry. Return the onion to the food processor.
4. Add 7 of the garlic cloves, the rosemary, oregano, lamb, salt, and pepper to the processor. Process until everything is well mixed into a paste, about 3 minutes. You may need to scrape the sides down a few times during this process.

5. Pack the meat mixture into a loaf pan. Put the loaf pan in the pan of water in the oven, and bake it until the internal temperature is 165°F, about 1 hour. Allow the meat to rest for 30 minutes.

6. Finely mince the remaining 1 clove garlic. In a small bowl, whisk together the Homemade Mayonnaise and the minced garlic.

7. Slice the meat into thin slices. Serve in a pita topped with the arugula, red onions, and garlic mayonnaise.

PER SERVING Calories: 516; Total Fat: 22g; Saturated Fat: 5g; Cholesterol: 110mg; Carbohydrates: 46g; Fiber: 6g; Protein: 40g

SPAGHETTI CARBONARA

Serves 4 / Prep time: 10 minutes / Cook time: 15 minutes

REINTRODUCING GLUTEN

This bacon and egg pasta is an Italian classic, and it's really easy to make. Use a whole-grain spaghetti to up the fiber intake.

NIGHTSHADE-FREE

NUT-FREE

QUICK & EASY

1 pound whole-grain spaghetti

6 slices bacon, cut into pieces

1 shallot, finely chopped

2 garlic cloves, minced

2 eggs, beaten

½ teaspoon sea salt

½ teaspoon freshly ground black pepper

2 tablespoons chopped fresh Italian parsley

1. In a large pot of boiling water, cook the pasta according to the package instructions. When done, drain and set aside.

2. Meanwhile, in a large sauté pan over medium-high heat, cook the bacon until it is crisp, about 6 minutes. Remove the bacon from the fat with a slotted spoon and set it aside to drain on a paper towel.

3. In the fat remaining from the bacon, cook the shallot until it is soft, about 4 minutes.

4. Add the garlic and cook, stirring constantly, until it is fragrant, about 30 seconds.

5. Reduce the heat to medium. Add the cooked pasta and reserved bacon to the pan and cook, stirring until it is warmed, about 2 minutes.

6. In a small bowl, whisk together the eggs, salt, and pepper. Take the pan off the heat, and pour the egg mixture into the pan. Stir constantly, until the egg cooks and the sauce thickens, about 1 minute more.

7. Stir in the parsley and serve.

PER SERVING Calories: 354; Total Fat: 15g; Saturated Fat: 5g; Cholesterol: 155mg; Carbohydrates: 33g; Fiber: 3g; Protein: 20g

PIZZA FRITTATA

Serves 4 / Prep time: 10 minutes / Cook time: 10 minutes

REINTRODUCING DAIRY

If you've missed pizza, you're in luck. This frittata takes the classic flavors of pizza and gives them back to you in a delicious egg dish. You can make this frittata ahead of time, cut it into wedges, and refrigerate them to reheat later. Feel free to replace the toppings suggested here with your own favorite pizza toppings.

¼ pound Italian Sausage (page 234)
4 ounces uncured pepperoni
4 ounces Canadian bacon
6 eggs, beaten
½ teaspoon garlic powder
1 teaspoon onion powder
¼ teaspoon sea salt
½ teaspoon dried oregano
¼ cup grated Parmesan cheese

NIGHTSHADE-FREE

NUT-FREE

MAKE-AHEAD

QUICK & EASY

1. Preheat the broiler to high.

2. In a large ovenproof baking pan over medium-high heat, cook the Italian Sausage, crumbling as you cook, until it browns, about 5 minutes.

3. Add the pepperoni and Canadian bacon, and cook to warm it for 1 minute more.

4. In a large bowl, whisk together the eggs, garlic powder, onion powder, salt, and oregano. Pour the mixture carefully over the meat in the pan, and reduce the heat to medium.

5. Cook without stirring until the eggs start to set, about 4 minutes.

6. Sprinkle the cheese over the top, and transfer the pan to the broiler. Broil until the top sets and the cheese starts to brown, another 3 to 5 minutes.

7. Cut into wedges and serve.

PER SERVING Calories: 284; Total Fat: 20g; Saturated Fat: 7g; Cholesterol: 294mg; Carbohydrates: 2g; Fiber 0g; Protein: 24g

CRUSTLESS MUSHROOM AND SWISS QUICHE

Serves 4 / Prep time: 20 minutes / Cook time: 45 minutes

REINTRODUCING DAIRY

NIGHTSHADE-
FREE

NUT-FREE

VEGETARIAN

MAKE-AHEAD

This quiche keeps really well. Just cut it into single servings and put it in a zipper bag. You can refrigerate the quiche for up to one week or freeze it for up to one year, and it reheats beautifully in the microwave. While the recipe calls for button mushrooms, feel free to use your favorites. My favorite mushrooms are chanterelles, which are available in the fall.

2 tablespoons coconut oil

1 onion, chopped

8 ounces sliced button mushrooms

6 eggs

¾ cup milk

½ teaspoon sea salt

¼ teaspoon freshly ground black pepper

½ teaspoon garlic powder

1 cup grated Swiss cheese

1. Preheat the oven to 350°F.

2. Grease a 9-inch square pan with coconut oil.

3. In a large sauté pan over medium-high heat, heat the coconut oil until it shimmers.

4. Add the onion and cook, stirring occasionally, until it is browned, about 6 minutes.

5. Add the mushrooms and cook, stirring occasionally, until they are soft, another 6 minutes.

6. Allow the mushrooms and onions to cool.

7. In a large bowl, whisk together the eggs, milk, salt, pepper, and garlic powder.

8. Fold in the cooled mushrooms, onions, and Swiss cheese.

9. Pour the mixture into the prepared pan. Bake until the quiche is set and browned, about 45 minutes.

Ingredient tip: For some extra iron and vitamins, add 2 cups of baby spinach to the mushrooms and onion as you cook them.

PER SERVING Calories: 303; Total Fat: 22g; Saturated Fat: 13g; Cholesterol: 274mg; Carbohydrates: 9g; Fiber: 1g; Protein: 19g

ITALIAN BURGERS STUFFED WITH MOZZARELLA

Serves 8 / Prep time: 20 minutes / Cook time: 20 minutes

REINTRODUCING DAIRY

NIGHTSHADE-FREE

MAKE-AHEAD

These juicy burger patties have more flavor than your typical hamburger. Serve them in a lettuce wrap topped with pesto mayonnaise. You can find fresh mozzarella in the specialty cheese section at the grocery store. It is typically packed in water.

FOR THE BURGERS

1 pound ground beef

1 pound Italian Sausage (page 234)

½ cup almond meal

1 egg, beaten

2 garlic cloves, minced

1 tablespoon Italian seasoning

¼ teaspoon sea salt

¼ teaspoon freshly ground black pepper

8 slices fresh mozzarella

8 large butter lettuce leaves

FOR THE PESTO MAYONNAISE

2 garlic cloves, minced

1 cup fresh basil leaves

¼ cup extra-virgin olive oil

¼ cup Parmesan cheese

¼ cup pine nuts

¾ cup Homemade Mayonnaise (page 229)

TO MAKE THE BURGERS

1. In a large bowl, mix together the ground beef, sausage, almond meal, egg, garlic, Italian seasoning, salt, and pepper.

2. Form the mixture into 16 thin patties. Place a slice of mozzarella on 8 of the patties, and then cover them with the 8 remaining patties. Seal the edges to make 8 stuffed patties.

3. Heat a large nonstick sauté pan over medium-high heat. Add the patties and cook until they are cooked through, about 7 minutes per side.

4. Use the butter lettuce as the buns.

TO MAKE THE PESTO MAYONNAISE

1. In the bowl of a food processor, process the garlic, basil, olive oil, Parmesan, and pine nuts until the pesto is finely chopped, about 1 minute.

2. In a small bowl, stir together the pesto and the Homemade Mayonnaise.

3. Serve with the burgers.

Substitution tip: If you are sensitive to nuts and seeds, you can leave out the almond meal in the burgers. It will result in a slightly denser burger. You should also leave out the pine nuts in the pesto and increase the Parmesan cheese to ½ cup.

PER SERVING Calories: 642; Total Fat: 48g; Saturated Fat: 14g; Cholesterol: 151mg; Carbohydrates: 9g; Fiber: 1g; Protein: 43g

CHICKEN AND EDAMAME SALAD

Serves 4 / Prep time: 15 minutes / Cook time: 0 minutes

REINTRODUCING SOY

Using a rotisserie chicken to make this tasty salad saves you time. You can use the carcass of the chicken to make some Slow Cooker Bone Broth (page 226), so don't throw it away. This salad will keep for up to three days in the refrigerator. It won't freeze well.

NIGHTSHADE-
FREE

NUT-FREE

MAKE-AHEAD

QUICK &
EASY

1 pound meat from a rotisserie chicken, cut into chunks

1 (14-ounce) package frozen edamame out of the pod, thawed and rinsed

1 celery stalk, chopped

6 scallions, thinly sliced

1 carrot, grated

¼ cup Homemade Mayonnaise (page 229)

Juice of 1 orange

Zest of ½ orange

2 tablespoons chopped fresh tarragon

½ teaspoon sea salt

¼ teaspoon freshly ground black pepper

1. In a large bowl, stir together the chicken, edamame, celery, scallions, and carrot.

2. In a small bowl, whisk together the Homemade Mayonnaise, orange juice, orange zest, tarragon, salt, and pepper.

3. Fold the dressing into the salad and serve.

PER SERVING Calories: 401; Total Fat: 15g; Saturated Fat: 3g; Cholesterol: 91mg; Carbohydrates: 21g; Fiber: 5g; Protein: 47g

COCONUT CURRY TOFU

Serves 4 / Prep time: 20 minutes / Cook time: 15 minutes

REINTRODUCING SOY

Use a firm tofu with this recipe for the right texture. You can use your favorite curry powder or curry blend. The recipe cooks really quickly in one pot. If you'd like a little more substance, serve it with a cup of Cauliflower "Rice" (page 231).

NIGHTSHADE-
FREE

NUT-FREE

VEGAN

2 tablespoons coconut oil

8 scallions, thinly sliced

8 ounces shiitake mushrooms, sliced

1 (14-ounce) can coconut milk

1½ teaspoons minced fresh ginger

1 teaspoon gluten-free soy sauce

1½ teaspoons curry powder

16 ounces extra-firm tofu, cut into ½-inch cubes

1 sweet potato, peeled and cut into ½-inch cubes

1. In a large pot over medium-high heat, heat the coconut oil until it shimmers. Add the scallions and mushrooms, and cook, stirring occasionally, until the mushrooms are browned, about 6 minutes.

2. Add the coconut milk, ginger, soy sauce, and curry powder, and bring the mixture to a simmer.

3. Add the tofu and sweet potatoes and cook, stirring frequently, until the potatoes are soft, about 15 minutes.

4. Serve warm.

PER SERVING Calories: 437; Total Fat: 36g; Saturated Fat: 28g; Cholesterol: 0mg; Carbohydrates: 24g; Fiber: 7g; Protein: 14g

TOFU AND VEGGIES IN ALMOND SAUCE

Serves 4 / Prep time: 20 minutes / Cook time: 10 minutes

REINTRODUCING SOY

VEGAN

QUICK &
EASY

A firm tofu is best for this recipe. If you like, you can make the tofu a bit firmer by putting it on a cutting board with one heavy-bottomed pan stacked on top of it for about 30 minutes to allow some of the extra water to drain away.

FOR THE TOFU AND VEGGIES

2 tablespoons coconut oil

½ onion, chopped

1 tablespoon fresh grated ginger

8 ounces shiitake mushrooms, sliced

2 cups broccoli florets

½ green bell pepper, chopped

16 ounces extra-firm tofu, cut into ½-inch cubes

3 garlic cloves, chopped

2 tablespoons gluten-free soy sauce

2 tablespoons rice wine vinegar

¼ teaspoon red pepper flakes

2 tablespoons arrowroot powder

FOR THE ALMOND SAUCE

1 garlic clove, minced

½ cup almond butter

2 tablespoons gluten-free soy sauce

¼ cup coconut milk

2 tablespoons chopped fresh cilantro

1 teaspoon fresh grated ginger

TO MAKE THE TOFU AND VEGGIES

1. In a large sauté pan over medium-high heat, heat the coconut oil until it shimmers. Add the onion and ginger and cook, stirring occasionally, until the onion is soft, about 5 minutes.

2. Add the mushrooms, broccoli, bell pepper, and tofu, and cook, stirring frequently, until it is cooked through, about 7 minutes more.

3. Add the garlic and cook, stirring constantly, until it is fragrant, about 30 seconds.

4. In a small bowl, whisk together the soy sauce, vinegar, red pepper flakes, and arrowroot. Add the mixture to the vegetables and cook, stirring constantly, until the sauce thickens, about 1 minute.

TO MAKE THE ALMOND SAUCE

1. In a small bowl, whisk together the garlic, almond butter, soy sauce, coconut milk, cilantro, and ginger until well combined.

2. Serve with the tofu and veggies.

PER SERVING Calories: 277; Total Fat: 16g; Saturated Fat: 10g; Cholesterol: 0mg; Carbohydrates: 21g; Fiber: 5g; Protein: 17g

QUINOA SALAD

Serves 6 / Prep time: 20 minutes / Cook time: 15 minutes /
Total time: 1 hour, 35 minutes

REINTRODUCING NON-GLUTEN GRAINS

*Always rinse quinoa before cooking to wash away any bitter flavors. Put
the quinoa in a fine-mesh sieve and run it under cool water. Allow it to drain
completely.*

2 cups Slow Cooker Bone Broth (page 226)

1 cup quinoa, uncooked

4 cups broccoli florets

2 cups sliced radishes

2 cups watercress

¼ cup extra-virgin olive oil

Juice of 2 lemons

Zest of 1 lemon

1 garlic clove, minced

½ teaspoon sea salt

2 tablespoons chopped fresh basil

1. In a large pan, bring the Slow Cooker Bone Broth to a boil.
2. Add the quinoa, and return it to a boil. Turn down the heat, and cover the pan. Cook on low for 15 minutes.
3. Take the pan off the heat, leaving it covered. Allow it to sit for 5 minutes more. Uncover and allow the quinoa to cool completely.
4. In a large bowl, stir together the cooled quinoa, broccoli florets, radish slices, and watercress.
5. In a small bowl, whisk together the olive oil, lemon juice, lemon zest, garlic, salt, and basil.
6. Toss the dressing with the salad and serve.

PER SERVING Calories: 222; Total Fat: 11g; Saturated Fat: 2g; Cholesterol: 0mg;
Carbohydrates: 24g; Fiber: 4g; Protein: 8g

FRIED RICE

Serves 6 / Prep time: 10 minutes / Cook time: 10 minutes

REINTRODUCING NON-GLUTEN GRAINS

The best thing about this fried rice is how quick and easy it is. You can find precooked white rice in the rice section at the grocery store. Alternately, you can order steamed rice from your local Asian restaurant.

2 tablespoons coconut oil

6 scallions, finely chopped

1 carrot, peeled and chopped

1 tablespoon ground ginger

3 garlic cloves, minced

4 eggs, beaten

4 cups cooked white rice

2 tablespoons coconut aminos

8 ounces cooked chicken from a rotisserie chicken

NIGHTSHADE-FREE

NUT-FREE

MAKE-AHEAD

QUICK & EASY

1. In a large sauté pan over medium-high heat, heat the coconut oil until it shimmers.

2. Add the scallions, carrot, and ginger, and cook, stirring occasionally, until the vegetables are soft, about 5 minutes.

3. Add the garlic and cook, stirring constantly, until it is fragrant, about 30 seconds.

4. Add the eggs and cook, stirring constantly, until the eggs set, about 2 minutes.

5. Add the rice, coconut aminos, and chicken. Cook, stirring constantly, until it is heated through, about 3 minutes more.

6. Serve warm.

Time-saving tip: Make this recipe even quicker by purchasing pre-chopped vegetables in the produce section or from your grocery store's salad bar.

PER SERVING Calories: 545; Total Fat: 8g; Saturated Fat: 5g; Cholesterol: 109mg; Carbohydrates: 102g; Fiber: 2g; Protein: 13g

OATMEAL "RISOTTO" with MUSHROOMS

Serves 4 / Prep time: 10 minutes / Cook time: 35 minutes

REINTRODUCING NON-GLUTEN GRAINS

Who says oatmeal is just for breakfast and cookies? This savory version of oatmeal is rich, flavorful, and deliciously satisfying. While it calls for cremini mushrooms, you can use any mushrooms that are in season.

NIGHTSHADE-FREE

NUT-FREE

MAKE-AHEAD

2 ounces dried porcini mushrooms

2 cups Slow Cooker Bone Broth (page 226)

1 cup steel-cut oats

2 tablespoons animal fat, such as lard

4 ounces pancetta, diced

1 onion, chopped

8 ounces cremini mushrooms, sliced

1 teaspoon dried thyme

½ teaspoon sea salt

¼ teaspoon freshly ground black pepper

1. In a large pot over high heat, bring the porcini mushrooms and Slow Cooker Bone Broth to a boil. Add the oats, and reduce the heat to medium. Simmer, stirring occasionally, for 25 minutes, until the oats are soft.

2. In a large sauté pan over medium-high heat, heat the fat until it shimmers. Add the pancetta and cook, stirring frequently, until it is crisp, about 5 minutes. Using a slotted spoon, remove the pancetta from the fat and set it aside.

3. Add the onions and cremini mushrooms to the sauté pan and cook, stirring occasionally, until the mushrooms are browned, about 7 minutes.

4. Add the pancetta, mushrooms and onions, thyme, salt, and pepper to the cooked oatmeal.

5. Cook, stirring frequently, for 5 minutes more, and serve.

PER SERVING Calories: 374; Total Fat: 20g; Saturated Fat: 7g; Cholesterol: 37mg; Carbohydrates: 27g; Fiber: 7g; Protein: 19g

THREE-BEAN SALAD

Serves 8 / Prep time: 10 minutes, plus 8 hours to chill

REINTRODUCING LEGUMES

The longer this salad sits, the more flavorful it gets as the beans soak up the vinaigrette. Be sure to drain and rinse the beans thoroughly before mixing them into the salad. Then, you can let the salad sit for up to a week in the refrigerator, which makes it a great weekday lunch.

1 (14-ounce) can kidney beans, drained and rinsed

1 (14-ounce) can garbanzo beans (chickpeas), drained and rinsed

1 (14-ounce) can green beans, drained and rinsed

1 red onion, finely chopped

1 celery stalk, thinly sliced

¼ cup extra-virgin olive oil

3 tablespoons red wine vinegar

1 teaspoon Dijon mustard

1 garlic clove, minced

1 teaspoon dried oregano

½ teaspoon sea salt

¼ teaspoon freshly ground black pepper

NIGHTSHADE-FREE

NUT-FREE

VEGAN

MAKE-AHEAD

QUICK & EASY

1. In a large bowl, mix the kidney beans, garbanzo beans, green beans, red onions, and celery.

2. In a small bowl, whisk together the olive oil, vinegar, mustard, garlic, oregano, salt, and pepper.

3. Pour the dressing over the salad, and toss to combine. Refrigerate for at least 8 hours before serving.

Substitution tip: You can replace the garbanzo and kidney beans with any other canned beans you enjoy, such as white beans or navy beans.

PER SERVING Calories: 426; Total Fat: 10g; Saturated Fat: 1g; Cholesterol: 0mg; Carbohydrates: 65g; Fiber: 19g; Protein: 22g

CANNELLINI AND ROSEMARY SOUP

Serves 6 / Prep time: 10 minutes / Cook time: 20 minutes

REINTRODUCING LEGUMES

This soup keeps really well in the refrigerator or freezer, so it's perfect for lunch or dinner. With cannellini beans, rosemary, and chicken, it has a delicious flavor that warms you up on chilly fall or winter evenings.

NIGHTSHADE-FREE

NUT-FREE

MAKE-AHEAD

QUICK & EASY

2 tablespoons animal fat, such as lard

1 onion, chopped

2 carrots, chopped

1 celery stalk, chopped

3 garlic cloves, minced

6 cups Slow Cooker Bone Broth (page 226)

2 (14-ounce) cans cannellini beans, drained and rinsed

8 ounces cooked chicken

2 teaspoons dried rosemary

1 teaspoon sea salt

¼ teaspoon freshly ground black pepper

1. In a large pot over medium-high heat, heat the fat until it shimmers.

2. Add the onion, carrots, and celery, and cook, stirring occasionally, until the vegetables are soft, about 6 minutes.

3. Add the garlic and cook, stirring constantly, until it is fragrant, about 30 seconds.

4. Add the Slow Cooker Bone Broth, beans, chicken, rosemary, salt, and pepper.

5. Simmer until the beans are warmed through, about 5 minutes more, and serve.

PER SERVING Calories: 346; Total Fat: 7g; Saturated Fat: 2g; Cholesterol: 33mg; Carbohydrates: 45g; Fiber: 18g; Protein: 28g

SLOW COOKER WHITE BEAN CHICKEN CHILI

Serves 8 / Prep time: 10 minutes / Cook time: 10 hours

REINTRODUCING LEGUMES

White bean chili makes a nice departure from darker chilies that have beef and red sauce. The beans and chicken have a delicate flavor that soaks in the spices. Of course, you can substitute any type of beans you like in this chili.

4 boneless, skinless chicken thighs, cut into ½-inch pieces

2 (14-ounce) cans white beans, drained and rinsed

1 red onion, chopped

1 jalapeño pepper, seeded and minced

4 garlic cloves, minced

1 tablespoon chili powder

½ teaspoon chipotle powder

½ teaspoon dried oregano

½ teaspoon ground cumin

1 teaspoon sea salt

2 cups Slow Cooker Bone Broth (page 226)

1. In the crock of a slow cooker, stir together the chicken, beans, onion, jalapeño, garlic, chili powder, chipotle powder, oregano, cumin, salt, and Slow Cooker Bone Broth. Cover the slow cooker, and set it on low.

2. Cook for 10 hours.

PER SERVING Calories: 484; Total Fat: 7g; Saturated Fat: 2g; Cholesterol: 62mg; Carbohydrates: 63g; Fiber: 16g; Protein: 45g

NUT-FREE

MAKE-AHEAD

QUICK & EASY

TEN TIPS FOR EATING OUT

When you're on a special diet, restaurant dining can be tricky. This is especially true when you must avoid common foods like gluten and dairy. I understand this completely. With celiac disease, even the slightest gluten contamination can leave me very sick. For a long time, I just avoided going to restaurants. While that saved me a lot of money, it wasn't a very practical strategy for the long term. Fortunately, I've learned some strategies that have really helped me with dining out, and they can help you stick to your plan as well.

1. Plan ahead.

If there's one thing I've learned, it's that planning ahead makes a huge difference. Whenever possible, I familiarize myself with the restaurant menu ahead of time and plan for what I will order. I even do this while I'm traveling, pulling up the restaurant menu on my smartphone to determine which items are "safe."

2. Talk to your server.

I used to hate "being that person." You know—the one in restaurants who has all sorts of picky requests. I discovered, though, that if I wanted to eat in restaurants without getting sick, I had to just get over it. I start the conversation by telling the server I have several food allergies. Using the word "allergy" is very important, because restaurants don't want to be liable for you having a reaction. Tell the server the foods you avoid, labeling them as allergies, and ask questions about how each item is prepared.

3. Establish rapport.

I've found that being super friendly and polite to my servers is very helpful. I let them know from the start how much I appreciate their recommendations, as well as their willingness to accommodate my food allergies. I also leave an excellent tip for the servers who work with me.

4. If possible, avoid busy times.

While this isn't always possible, especially if you're on the road, going out to eat at times that are not the restaurant's peak times is very helpful. Your server and the chef will have more time to talk with you, accommodate your requests, and make recommendations when they aren't slammed with customers. That means I eat a lot of early bird or late meals, but it makes my experience in restaurants so much easier.

5. Have a few go-to menu items.

If you eat in certain restaurants a lot, such as casual dining or fast food restaurants, do your research well ahead of time and know exactly which menu items will work on your diet. That way, you know exactly where you can dine and what you can order when you're in a hurry.

6. Choose simple menu items.

The simpler a menu item is, the less likely it is to contain hidden foods you can't eat. So a steak and steamed vegetables will be much more likely to be "clean" than a soup or a stew.

7. Ask questions.

Don't be afraid to ask questions about menu items. When I'm in a restaurant, I pepper the server with questions about menu items I am considering. I ask about what's in the seasoning blends, whether they marinate meats, and what seasonings they put on their foods. It helps me make more informed decisions, and I am less likely to eat something that's not good for me.

8. Call ahead.

If I know I am going to a restaurant for a family gathering where I haven't chosen the location myself, I call ahead. When I call, I tell them I am coming for a family gathering and I have some severe food allergies. I ask if they have an allergens menu, and I ask where I can access it ahead of time. I also ask if they will be able to accommodate my allergies. If not, I eat ahead of time and have a beverage while at the restaurant.

9. When in doubt, order something else.

If your server can't tell you to your satisfaction whether a menu item contains the foods you are avoiding, your best strategy is to order something else. Always err on the side of caution.

10. Order off-menu.

I have found that most restaurants will be willing to make you a few simple off-menu items. These include salads with oil and vinegar, steamed vegetables, and a simple grilled piece of meat. Request that they use only salt and pepper for seasoning and they avoid cooking with butter or oils other than olive oil.

APPENDIX B
SHOPPING RESOURCES

I discovered when I switched to my current way of eating that I had to learn to shop in a new way. I live in a very small community with tiny grocery stores, and I wasn't having a lot of luck finding the foods I needed. Because of that, I learned new strategies for shopping that made things much easier for me. Hopefully, these resources will help you as well.

Organic Local Produce

If you don't live near a grocery store with a killer organic produce section, such as Whole Foods, then you'll probably need to find a few places that will suit your needs.

Farmers' Markets and CSAs

Farmers' markets offer wonderful seasonal produce from organic and conventional farmers. Because the produce offered is usually from within a hundred miles, it tends to be extremely fresh and flavorful.

CSA—or community supported agriculture—is another good, and affordable, way to receive fresh produce several months out of the year. With a CSA program, you pay a monthly or seasonal fee for a weekly box of fresh produce from a local farmer. Being part of a CSA allows you to learn to work with seasonal fruits and vegetables you may never have tried before. Likewise, the ingredients you get in your weekly CSA box are extremely fresh, making them a delicious addition to your food plan.

Local Harvest (localharvest.org) is a great resource for finding farmers' markets and CSAs. It has a searchable database that helps you find organic produce in your area.

Co-Ops, Farm Stands, and Produce Markets

Natural food co-ops are an affordable way to find local organic produce. Visit the Co-Op Directory (coopdirectory.org) to search for co-ops near you.

Farm stands offer a diversity of freshly picked produce. The Farmstand App (farmstandapp.com) for your smartphone is a great way to find nearby stands, no matter where you are.

Local produce markets specialize in selling an array of regional organic vegetables. If you always drive past your local produce market and think about stopping but never do (which is what I did for years), pop in and see what they have to offer.

Organic Pastured Meats

While I do still occasionally eat conventional meats, I try to stick with meats that come from pastured and naturally raised animals. In beef, you'll find this referred to as "grass-fed." With poultry, you may find it called "free-range." With pork, it's usually referred to as "pastured," while fish is "wild-caught." All of these labels mean that the meats are allowed to graze on the foods they would naturally eat in the wild—grasses, seeds, grubs, etc.—as opposed to being fed grains in a feed lot.

Organic meats are hormone-free and antibiotic-free. They also are fed food that doesn't contain any pesticides, chemicals, antibiotics, or hormones.

Not all organic meat is pastured, and not all pastured meat is organic. Whenever possible, try to eat meats that are organic and pastured. Unless you have a great natural market in your area, you may have difficulty locating these meats.

EatWild.Com

This Internet database helps you locate local ranchers offering organic pastured meats and eggs. It is searchable by zip code. While many of the ranchers sell the meat in bulk, others sell at local farmers' markets, have stores on their property, or sell meats by the piece instead of by the whole animal or side.

US Wellness Meats

This online meat retailer has an excellent selection of pastured animal products, including beef, pork, duck, buffalo (bison), poultry, and wild-caught fish. They ship in freezer containers with ice using two-day shipping, and the meat arrives frozen. The meat is high in quality. On Mondays, they also receive a shipment of sugar-free bacon and sugar-free pork sausage. While it goes quickly, it's worth the effort if you can grab some. Visit GrasslandBeef.com.

Tendergrass Farms

While their selection isn't as broad as US Wellness Meats' inventory, Tendergrass Farms has a nice selection of beef, chicken, and pork. They also sell sugar-free bacon, sugar-free breakfast sausage, sugar-free hot dogs, and sugar-free Italian sausage, so if you don't want to make your own, it's a great resource. Visit GrassFedBeef.org.

REFERENCES

Abbas, Abul K., Lichtman, Andrew H., and Pillai, Shiv. *Basic Immunology: Functions and Disorders of the Immune System*, 4th ed. Philadelphia: Saunders, 2012.

American Autoimmune Related Diseases Association. "Autoimmune Statistics." Accessed June 15, 2014. http://www.aarda.org/autoimmune-information/autoimmune-statistics/.

Arizona Center for Advanced Medicine. "Leaky Gut—Real or Imaginary?" Accessed February 21, 2015. http://arizonaadvancedmedicine.com/leaky-gut-real-imaginary/.

Bhuyan, Ashok K., Sarma, Dipti, and Saikia, Uma K. "Selenium and the thyroid: A close-knit connection." *Indian Journal of Endocrinology and Metabolism* 16, suppl 2 (December 2012): S354–S355.

Blum, Susan, MD. *The Immune System Recovery Plan*. New York: Scribner, 2013.

Boelaert, Kristien, Newby, Paul R., et al. "Prevalence and Relative Risk of Other Autoimmune Diseases in Subjects with Autoimmune Thyroid Disease." *American Journal of Medicine* 123, no. 2 (February 2010): 183.e1–183.e9.

Celiac Central. "Celiac Disease: Fast Facts." Accessed February 21, 2015. http://www.celiaccentral.org/celiac-disease/facts-and-figures/.

———. "Non-Celiac Gluten Sensitivity." Accessed February 21, 2015. http://www.celiaccentral.org/non-celiac-gluten-sensitivity/.

Center for Food Safety. "About Genetically Engineered Foods." Accessed February 21, 2015. http://www.centerforfoodsafety.org/issues/311/ge-foods/about-ge-foods#.

De Punder, Karin, and Leo Pruimboom. "The Dietary Intake of Wheat and other Cereal Grains and Their Role in Inflammation." *Nutrients* 5, no. 3 (March 2013): 771–787.

Environmental Working Group. "EWG's 2014 Shopper's Guide to Pesticides in Produce." Accessed February 21, 2015. http://www.ewg.org/foodnews/.

Johns Hopkins Medical Institutions, Autoimmune Disease Research Center. "Frequently Asked Questions." Accessed February 21, 2015. http://autoimmune.pathology.jhmi.edu/faqs.cfm.

Kasai, M., Nosaka, N., Maki, H., et al. "Comparison of diet-induced thermogenesis of foods containing medium- versus long-chain triacylglycerols." *Journal of Nutritional Science and Vitaminology* 48, no. 6 (2002): 536–40.

King Corn. "About *King Corn*." Accessed February 21, 2015. http://www.kingcorn.net/.

Kresser, Chris. "Iodine for Hypothyroidism: Crucial Nutrient or Harmful Toxin?" ChrisKresser.com. Accessed February 21, 2015. http://chriskresser.com/iodine-for-hypothyroidism-like-gasoline-on-a-fire.

———. "The Role of Vitamin D Deficiency in Thyroid Disorders." ChrisKresser.com. Accessed February 21, 2015. http://chriskresser.com/the-role-of-vitamin-d-deficiency-in-thyroid-disorders.

Linus Pauling Institute. "Zinc." Oregon State University. Accessed February 21, 2015. http://lpi.oregonstate.edu/infocenter/minerals/zinc/.

Masterjohn, Christopher. "New Evidence of Synergy Between Vitamins A and D: Protection Against Autoimmune Diseases." Weston A. Price Foundation. Accessed February 21, 2015. http://www.westonaprice.org/blogs/cmasterjohn/new-evidence-of-synergy-between-vitamins-a-and-d-protection-against-autoimmune-diseases/.

Mayo Clinic Staff. "Hashimoto's Disease: Symptoms." Mayo Clinic. Accessed February 21, 2015. http://www.mayoclinic.org/diseases-conditions/hashimotos-disease/basics/symptoms/con-20030293.

National Endocrine and Metabolic Disease Information Service. "Hashimoto's Disease." Accessed February 21, 2015. http://www.endocrine.niddk.nih.gov/pubs/hashimoto/.

———. "Pregnancy and Thyroid Disease." Accessed February 21, 2015. http://www.endocrine.niddk.nih.gov/pubs/pregnancy/#postpartum.

National Institutes of Health. "TSH Test." MedlinePlus. Accessed February 21, 2015. http://www.nlm.nih.gov/medlineplus/ency/article/003684.htm.

Natural Resources Defense Council. "Consumer Guide to Mercury in Fish." Accessed February 21, 2015. http://www.nrdc.org/health/effects/mercury/guide.asp.

Pick, Marcelle, OB/GYN, NP. "Causes of Inflammation." Women to Women. Accessed February 21, 2015. https://www.womentowomen.com/inflammation/causes-of-inflammation/.

Teicholz, Nina. *The Big Fat Surprise.* New York: Simon & Schuster, 2014.

US Department of Health and Human Services. "Hashimoto's Disease." Women'sHealth.gov. Accessed February 21, 2015. http://www.womenshealth.gov/publications/our-publications/fact-sheet/hashimoto-disease.html.

USDA Economic Research Service. "Adoption of Genetically Engineered Crops in the U.S." Accessed February 21, 2015. http://www.ers.usda.gov/data-products/adoption-of-genetically-engineered-crops-in-the-us/recent-trends-in-ge-adoption.aspx.

WebMD. "Depression, the Thyroid, and Hormones." Accessed February 21, 2015. http://www.webmd.com/depression/guide/depression-the-thyroid-and-hormones.

Weil, Andrew, MD. "Q&A Library: What Is Leaky Gut?" Accessed February 21, 2015. http://www.drweil.com/drw/u/QAA361058/what-is-leaky-gut.html.

INDEX